THE
T-FACTOR
DIET

Also by Martin Katahn, PhD,
and published by Bantam Books

THE ROTATION DIET

THE ROTATION DIET COOKBOOK

(with Terri Katahn)

T-FACTOR diet

MARTIN KATAHN PhD

BANTAM BOOKS
TORONTO · NEW YORK · LONDON · SYDNEY · AUCKLAND

THE T-FACTOR DIET
A BANTAM BOOK 0 553 40065 7

Originally published in Great Britain by
Bantam Press, a division of Transworld Publishers Ltd

PRINTING HISTORY
Bantam Press edition published 1989
Bantam Books edition published 1990

Bantam Books are published by Transworld Publishers
Ltd., 61–63 Uxbridge Road, Ealing, London W5 5SA, in
Australia by Transworld Publishers (Australia) Pty. Ltd.,
15–23 Helles Avenue, Moorebank, NSW 2170, and in New
Zealand by Transworld Publishers (N.Z.) Ltd., Cnr. Moselle
and Waipareira Avenues, Henderson, Auckland.

Printed and bound in Great Britain by
Cox & Wyman Ltd., Reading, Berks.

CONTENTS

ACKNOWLEDGEMENTS

This book and the research in the Vanderbilt Weight Management Program that confirms the validity and usefulness of its concepts are made possible by many people. I would like to express my appreciation to:

Jamie Pope-Cordle, MS, RD, for designing the basic menus and analysing nutrient values, developing many of the recipes, helping to lead the T-Factor research groups, supplying much of the material for the chapter on childhood and adolescent nutrition, and for her comments and suggestions on the manuscript.

James O. Hill, PhD, for developing Vanderbilt University's calorimetry chamber, for designing our metabolic research programme, and for reading critically and commenting on the manuscript.

David G. Schlundt, PhD, for directing the Vanderbilt Weight Management Research Program and for helping to design and evaluate the clinical research on which the T-Factor Diet is based.

Tracy Sbrocco for developing the nutrient databank for the Fat and Fibre Counter.

Harriet Simpkins for coordinating groups, supplying information and encouragement to the thousands of people who have telephoned the Vanderbilt Program for help from all over the United States during the past few years, and being ready to jump in and do anything we need done whenever we need her help.

Veronica Petta, MA, *Family Circle* home economist and nutritionist, for developing a batch of delicious, nutritious recipes for the T-Factor Diet.

Terri Katahn for helping to develop the menus and recipes,

supplying the helpful information contained in the introductions to all the recipe sections, and providing critical comments and suggestions during the writing of the manuscript.

Enid Katahn for undying love and patience during the unavoidable stressful periods that arise with every book I write – the final stages always seem to occur at the end of a fall semester at the University, and while I am trying to complete several other projects.

Mary Bomar, who is really Enid's Personal Representative, for tending the home office and doing everything from analysing nutrient data to booking concerts and walking the dog when necessary.

Joyce Weingartner for her excellent bread recipes, which I include once again in the book.

ESHA Research for the Food Processor II Nutrient and Diet Analysis System which supplies the programme we use to analyse our menus and recipes and especially to Elizabeth Geltz for always being Johnny-on-the-spot whenever I have a question.

Starling Lawrence, my editor at W. W. Norton, with whom I've worked so closely on five books going on six, for making it his business to know as much about the field I work in as possible, which in turn enables him to help me clarify the often complex concepts with which I work.

Artie and Richard Pine, my literary agents, for their help in attending to all the matters authors are so poor at, but mostly for friendship and enthusiasm for my work during the many years we have worked together.

All my other friends and helpers at W. W. Norton, and also Doug Stallings, Ralph Kirkland and the entire staff at the Tandy Computer Center and the Tandy Area Training and Support Group for their attention to my personal needs as well as to the needs of the research group in the Weight Management Program at Vanderbilt University.

Again, thank you all very much.

THE T-FACTOR DIET

CHAPTER ONE

INTRODUCTION

A calorie is a calorie is a calorie. Right?

WRONG!

The T-Factor Diet is based on recent scientific discoveries in the fields of biochemistry and physiology that reveal major differences in the way our bodies process, utilize and store the calories in our food. These studies also show how you can activate your body's innate, natural fat-burning potential and melt away excess body fat without actually cutting back on your total caloric intake.

First, research in the biochemistry field shows that many of our old ideas about the caloric value of foods to the human body were wrong. All calories are not the same to the human body. When it comes to being fat and overweight, it's primarily the fat calories that count, *not* the carbohydrate and protein calories.

Second, research in the field of physiology shows that many forms of physical activity used by overweight people in their quest for weight reduction, *in combination with the typical mix of nutrients in their diets*, can have little or no impact on their stores of body fat. While the research shows how to maximize the fat-burning power of exercise, it also explains how certain common combinations of exercise and diet can work against you and actually encourage the transformation of dietary fat to body fat.

The two lines of research that have inspired this book show that there is a particular combination of diet and physical activity that can lead you to a permanent reduction in body fat, *without cutting calories and without counting them.*

You will find that combination in the T-Factor Diet.

The T-Factor Diet is based on concepts that are going to revolutionize our thinking about the metabolism of energy in the human body as well as about weight management. Obviously, such claims require an explanation. Here is a brief summary of the scientific background; I will furnish more details in Chapter Two.

In the laboratory, when the caloric value of foods is measured, all calories are by definition equal. In the measurement of the energy of foods, a calorie* is the amount of heat it takes to raise the temperature of 1 kilogram of water 1 degree Celsius. Calories are measured in the laboratory by burning carefully measured portions of food in special instruments which in turn measure the amount of energy released. Until a few years ago, most experts considered that the human body extracted the energy from fat, carbohydrate, and protein with about equal efficiency. By this I mean that when we measured certain amounts of carbohydrate, protein, or fatty foods in the laboratory, and found that each contained 100 calories, we assumed that the human body also extracted 100 calories from those quantities and that the entire 100 calories would be available either for sustaining basal metabolic processes† or powering physical activity.

To use some actual examples: As measured in the laboratory, we assumed that 100 calories' worth of carbohydrate foods such as apples, carrots, potatoes and whole-grain bread and 100 calories' worth of fat or fatty foods such as butter, margarine, fried potatoes and sausages *each supplied the same amount of energy – 100 calories – for activity or metabolic functions*.

THIS IS FALSE!

A hundred calories of baked potatoes and 100 calories of chips are not equal, *except* in the laboratory! They have a very different impact on the human body.

The human body extracts and accumulates much more usable energy from fat than from any other nutrient. In addition, the body seems far, *far* more efficient at converting dietary fat into body fat than it is at converting carbohydrate or protein into body fat. Indeed, the differences in the way your body metabolizes fat com-

---

* When used as a measure of energy in food, the word *calorie* was originally capitalized or referred to as a kilocalorie. It was equal to 1000 'small' calories as used in the field of chemistry, where it is equal to the heat required to raise the temperature of 1 gram of water 1 degree, from 15 to 16 degrees Celsius.

† Basal metabolic processes: those maintenance functions that are essential to life, such as vital cellular activity, the circulation of blood, respiration etc. The basal metabolic rate is the energy required to maintain these functions in a fasting, resting organism.

pared with protein and carbohydrate are so great that, except for a small percentage of people who suffer from metabolic abnormality, YOU CAN'T GET FAT EXCEPT BY EATING FAT! 　　　.

And the precise way in which you get fat is by taking in more fat in your daily diet than you are burning up in the fuel mixture that keeps you alive each day.

I am going to present the facts behind these statements and explain them in full detail in Chapter Two and, for all people who fall within the range of normal metabolism, I make this promise:

The T-Factor Diet will turn on your body's innate, hidden potential for melting off excess body fat. If you stick with the T-Factor formula for the control of fat intake that I'll give you in Chapter Three, you will be able completely to satisfy your appetite and you will still lose weight painlessly and easily.

DO YOU HAVE TO CUT CALORIES TO LOSE WEIGHT?

It's traditional nutritional doctrine and, indeed, it seems only logical that: If you want to lose weight you have to cut your caloric intake, and if you want to maintain your weight loss after you've lost weight you have to consume fewer calories for ever. This logic is based on the belief that energy in the human being follows a simple rule: A given caloric intake yields a predictable surplus or deficit in fat storage depending on the amount of energy expended in daily life. Thus, to lose weight you have to unbalance the energy equation so that calories 'in' are fewer than calories 'out'.

The research to which I have already referred has shattered this logic and this belief. The total number of calories you eat may be less important than the source of those calories. As I said earlier, if you have surplus fat on your body, you are probably eating too much fat, not necessarily too many calories. In fact, the reason that most overweight people are overweight is that they eat *four or five times more fat than is essential, and about twice as much as is necessary to make a tasty, healthy, lifelong weight-maintenance diet.*

Of course, all health professionals are encouraging us to eat less fat – as the United States Surgeon General, Dr C. Everett Koop, recently pointed out, fat is Western society's greatest nutritional hazard. Why is it, however, that all this advice and exhortation is only marginally successful?

Let's make it personal! What about you? If you're one of the majority of the people in the Western world who are still consuming too much fat – the fat that's making you fat, and possibly contributing to premature heart disease and other ills – why haven't you followed this advice and cut back to desirable levels?

Believe me, there is no need to feel guilty about your preference for fatty foods. If you crave prime cuts of meat, fried foods, rich sauces and tasty desserts, it's not a moral issue. It's a biological issue. And I will explain all of this in Chapter Ten, with the hope of helping you to combat a perfectly normal predisposition that kept primitive humans alive when they faced periodic food shortages, but which does not serve you well in a society where rich foods are continually and easily available.

We must all face the fact that fat makes many foods, including many carbohydrate and protein foods, *taste better*! That's why so many of us choose to have chips and chops rather than baked or boiled potato and the lean flank of beef.

But there are ways of dealing effectively with our innate liking for fat and, for that matter, with our innate liking for sweet-tasting things as well. All of us in the Vanderbilt Weight Management Program have worked very hard on the T-Factor Diet to create a *livable* diet as well as a *workable* diet. I say this because just about any semi-starvation, reduced-calorie diet will *work temporarily* when it comes to losing weight; the real issue is, can you *live* with it?

Yes, you are going to have to change – you can't continue to do precisely as you have been doing in the way of diet and exercise and expect any change in the ease with which you manage your weight. But the T-Factor Diet can succeed for you where other diets have failed because, in addition to its fat-burning potential, it gets you off the ersatz, artificial products that research shows are little, if any, help in weight control. We are going to return to the foods that are much more satisfying to the human appetite, including the genuine, natural fats, oils and sweeteners.

I promise you a satisfying diet as well as a healthier diet. And, of course, it's going to solve your weight-management problems. As the saying goes, 'Try it – you'll like it!'

WHAT ABOUT EXERCISE?

I know I am going to surprise those of you who are familiar with my previous work on obesity with the following statement because I am such a strong proponent of physical fitness as a key to weight management, and I continue to be a strong proponent, but:

Yes! You can reduce your body fat without additional exercise by following the nutritional principles of the T-Factor Diet. I am very pleased to be able to say this, because, for the first time, there appears to be real hope for people who suffer from limitations in their ability to be active.

But I want to emphasise that the healthiest way to permanent weight management, *and the easiest and quickest*, is through a combination of the T-Factor Diet and its associated T-Factor forms of physical activity. Besides, physical activity has a special impact on our self-esteem and psychological well-being that cannot be matched by any other change in a sedentary person's lifestyle.

WHAT TO EXPECT IN THIS BOOK

In the next chapter (Chapter Two) I will explain what the T-Factor is and summarise the scientific research that led to the development of the T-Factor Diet and how it works. It is the healthiest diet there is for all normal people and you do not have to cut calories to burn off your unhealthy excess fat.*

And then we won't waste time: In Chapter Three I'll explain each of the principles of the T-Factor Diet fully and simply. If you are the kind of person who wants to just sit back and watch as the fat gradually falls off, there will be no calorie counting and no need to follow fixed menus unless you want my specific recommendations. Your excess fat will simply and naturally melt away, that is, be burned as fuel, until your body establishes a new equilibrium with the minimum of fat storage that was meant for you by Mother Nature. Because I am interested in helping you to eat a nutritious diet, I will, however, give suggestions for several basic breakfasts, lunches and dinners. I also include three weeks of specific daily menus. I want to show you that exactly the same principles apply to permanent weight management as to weight loss – *no more on-and-off diets*!

In Chapter Four I will present some personal experiences and hints from people who have been following the T-Factor Diet and who have permanently incorporated it into their lifestyle – including myself.

Although I hope you realize from your own past experience that the race may not go to the hare but to the tortoise, I know that some of you – especially those who have more than a few pounds to lose –

---

* Because the research is so new and has to date appeared only in scientific journals and has not been incorporated into nutrition textbooks, I present a much more in-depth and detailed discussion, with references, in Appendix A.

are in a hurry. I was when I lost my own excess 5 stone (34 kg) some twenty-six years ago. So long as you use a quick-loss plan that incorporates the principles you must incorporate permanently into your diet, a quick-loss plan need not be counterproductive and need not encourage a quick regaining of lost weight (as so many quick-loss plans do). It's really a matter of temperament and personal choice.

The Quick Melt plan, which I present in Chapter Five, is for those of you who want a safe head start on your weight-management programme. If you are considerably overweight, the Quick Melt can take off up to a pound a day. In contrast with the basic T-Factor Diet, the Quick Melt plan is calorie-reduced in order to pull extra fat from your fat cells. To make sure you are eating well during your Quick Melt, I present twenty-one days of sample menus. Incorporated in these menus are six special recipes developed by Ms Veronica Petta, MA, *Family Circle* home economist and nutritionist, specifically for the T-Factor Diet. I think they are delicious and that they will appeal to you.

If you choose to start with the Quick Melt, stick with it for three weeks. Then, if you have more weight to lose, use either the principles or the sample menus in Chapter Three to continue to your weight-loss goal. *You do not have to continue to cut calories to burn off excess body fat, and the sooner you begin to incorporate T-Factor principles and practice into your permanent eating plan WITHOUT cutting calories, the more certain you are of lifelong success.*

After you have been on a reduced-calorie diet, there is always the danger of a rapid gain should you increase calories too quickly. Chapter Five closes with transitional menus that will prevent your regaining the weight you have lost when you switch to maintenance after using the Quick Melt.

In Chapter Six I present many recipes to show you that the diet I am recommending is truly something you can live with for the rest of your life. Some of these recipes come from my own household, others from the director of nutrition of the Vanderbilt Weight Management Program, Ms Jamie Pope-Cordle, MS, RD, and others were developed by Ms Veronica Petta at *Family Circle* magazine. Still others demonstrate how participants in the Vanderbilt Weight Management Program responded to the challenge of modifying their own favourite dishes to fit the principles of the diet. Before being included in this book all recipes were repeatedly tested and, in addition to being delicious, are designed to serve as an education. I want to show you how to use T-Factor principles to prepare everything from soup to nuts, including your own favourites. I want everyone in your family to be happy about the changes you are making. Two things are certain: If you don't like what I'm encouraging you to do you will find it hard to stay with it, and if everyone in your family feels as though you're forcing *them* to go on a diet just because *you're* trying to lose weight, you're not going to get much co-operation.

Going on to my recommendations for physical activity in Chapter Seven, I will explain why some kinds of exercise do so little to help with weight control and how some forms of exercise, in combination with the typical Western diet, may actually encourage your body to gain fat. I will, of course, describe an activity pro-gramme that can make sure your body fat is at its healthiest, lowest minimum.

In Chapter Eight I will explain how psychological factors can play a key role in maintaining your motivation for physical activity. Our research shows that physical activity contributes more to the development of a positive self-concept than does weight loss itself.

With the help of Ms Pope-Cordle I have prepared a special chapter (Chapter Nine) on childhood and adolescent nutrition. Here I will explain how to help overweight children lose weight without going on a diet. Of course, even if your children are not overweight, the way to prevent weight problems in later life is to develop healthy eating and activity habits early in life.

In Chapter Ten I'll discuss some important myths and mis-understandings about obesity. I'll explain the likely origins of carbohydrate cravings and why we tend to have a preference for fatty foods. I'll also explain the real meaning of the term *set point* and how you can control it.

In order to help guarantee your success in losing weight, this book includes a fat-gram counter in Appendix C. If you really want to know how much fat you are eating, on which your body's fat storage depends, all you need to do is count your fat grams. When you reach the limit, you can eat just about anything you want if you are hungry, but it must *not* contain additional fat! The counter also includes the values of dietary fibre because the consumption of fibre can help assure that you obtain the maximum fat-burning impact of the T-Factor Diet, as well as a number of other health benefits.

HOW IS THE T-FACTOR DIET AN IMPROVEMENT OVER THE ROTATION DIET AND ANY OTHER WEIGHT-LOSS DIET?

The Rotation Diet was designed in 1984–5 by my colleagues and me in the Vanderbilt Weight Management Program to help people lose weight quickly without encountering the metabolic slowdown that often accompanies quick losses. It's a good, fast weight-loss diet that has helped millions of people lose weight. Our research results show that about 25 per cent of the people have lost weight permanently, and at least half of the users are remaining physically more active than before.

That's an excellent record, but the scientific discoveries that led to the development of the T-Factor Diet have now provided a way to improve on it. I will discuss the improvements in detail when I compare it with the Quick Melt in Chapter Five. In brief, the T-Factor Diet is more nutritious, easier to follow, has a much greater variety of foods and does not require low-calorie dieting for a quick loss. In particular, I'm concerned with the maintenance of weight loss, and while the Rotation Diet has done extremely well, it is a calorie-based and calorie-restricted diet. We now know the essential role that dietary fat plays in obesity, and that the key to permanent weight control has less to do with calories than with the fat in your diet. When people fail to keep their weight off after losing it on any diet, it's because they begin to consume more fat than they can burn off each day. When you fully understand this point and learn to incorporate its practical application into your own diet, you will never have a weight problem again.

WHAT'S IN STORE FOR YOU ON THE T-FACTOR DIET

'I can't believe I'm eating like this and losing weight!'

This is the most frequent comment that people on the T-Factor Diet make from Day 1. I wish I didn't have to call the T-Factor Diet a 'diet' because of the calorie-cutting associations that people make to that word. YOU ARE NOT GOING ON A DIET TO LOSE WEIGHT.

You are not going to be cutting calories or counting them.

Except for fat, you are going to be eating just about as much of everything as you want.

'I'm never hungry! There's always something good to eat!'

That's another frequent comment made by people on the T-Factor Diet.

From the very beginning you will be losing weight *and* eating delicious food according to the principles that will make it easy for you to maintain ideal weight for life. No more on-and-off diets. No more deprivation. No more obsessions with food. No more guilt

8

feelings. And no more wild desires to binge that can follow constant restraint.

I'll say it once again and then let you find out for yourself:

There is always something good to eat on the T-Factor Diet. You can lose weight and you can keep it off, and YOU'LL NEVER GO HUNGRY AGAIN!

CHAPTER TWO

THE THIN-FACTOR: THE SCIENTIFIC BACKGROUND OF THE T-FACTOR DIET*

The T-Factor is your THIN-Factor!

Essentially, the term 'T-Factor' refers to the energy-using processes by which your body turns food into fuel and burns fuel during exercise. These natural processes, labelled in the scientific field with unusual terms like 'thermic' and 'thermogenesis', can be harnessed to help you lose weight. I've grouped all these processes under the term *T-Factor* (the 'T' being the first letter of the words thermic and thermogenesis) and I'm going to explain why and how you can maximize your T-Factor so that you can actually eat more and weigh less! This is not an idle claim. Here's how it works.

There are three aspects to the T-Factor:

1. *The Thermic Effect of Food*. It takes energy to get energy! Your body burns up a certain number of calories simply turning the protein, carbohydrate and fat in your food into the form your body needs to stay alive and keep moving. *The amount of calories required in the conversion process is different for protein, carbohydrate and fat.*

2. *Adaptive Thermogenesis*. Your body also has the ability to adapt to changing circumstances. It can either *conserve* or *waste* a certain number of calories while it's turning your food into fuel and performing all the other functions necessary to life.

In its conservation mode, the metabolic processes are slow or sluggish. The body switches to conservation mode and slows down to protect a person against fat and protein loss in times of famine,

---

* In this chapter I present the conclusions from the most important research that led to the development of the T-Factor Diet. The actual studies are discussed in detail and referenced in Appendix A.

but, when plenty of food is available, this slowdown leads to easy weight gain.

In its wasteful mode your body's metabolic rate speeds up; the wasteful mode is nature's way of preventing weight gain and keeping people thin.

Without realizing it, however, overweight people keep their bodies in the conservation mode with an unwise choice of foods, going on and off diets, and, often, a lack of exercise. Obviously, if you want to lose weight and never regain it, you want to rev up and waste fuel. Fortunately, as you will soon discover, turning on your wasteful mode by speeding up your metabolism is good for your health as well as for your spirits and energy level.

3. *The Thermic Effect of Exercise.* Quick, explosive physical movements are powered by your body's carbohydrate energy stores, while sustained repetitive movements use primarily fat. This is why certain kinds of activity tend to be better for losing weight than others. We'll talk more about the T-Factor Exercise Programme in Chapter Seven.

You can take advantage of your body's natural fat-burning T-Factor in a number of ways, from how your body turns food into fuel to how it stores and burns fuel.

HOW THE BODY TURNS FOOD INTO FUEL

Until quite recently, experts in this field of nutrition assumed that the energy in different food sources, that is, protein, carbohydrate and fat, was extracted with about equal efficiency. Thus, if we overate on *any* source, all the surplus energy would end up in our fat cells. Calories contained in carbohydrate foods would make you just as fat as calories from fatty foods. Recent research in the area of biochemistry is about to revolutionise our views about how energy is extracted from the different foods and used by our bodies.

This new biochemical research has shown more clearly than ever that IT'S THE FAT IN YOUR DIET THAT MAKES YOU FAT.

This statement probably comes as no surprise to you, at least in part.

Anyone who has ever been on a diet knows that they must keep away from fatty foods, including fried foods and rich desserts. But what about grains, breads, potatoes, pasta, beans, rice and all those other starchy foods? How about those high-calorie natural sweets like dried fruits? Do we have to cut back on those foods in order to lose weight?

The answer is NO! Carbohydrate foods, including starchy foods

11

and dried fruits, actually turn on your T-Factor and help you to stay thin. Protein also turns on your T-Factor, but animal protein is often found together with a great deal of fat, and a diet high in protein is not recommended.

How do protein and carbohydrates affect your T-Factor? Why is it virtually impossible to get fat, or stay fat, when you follow the low-fat dietary guidelines in the T-Factor Diet?

Here are the facts:

1. First of all, protein is not a major factor in weight regulation. Within the normal range found in the typical Western diet, all the energy contained in the protein is burned in our daily fuel mixture and none is converted for fat storage. Indeed, it takes 25 per cent of the energy contained in protein just to transform it into the form our bodies need, so only 75 per cent is available for building and repairing cells and other metabolic functions.

2. Fat is another story. It takes hardly any energy at all to convert fat into a source of fuel for our bodies. A whopping 97 per cent of the calories in fat can be placed in permanent storage just where you don't want it if you overeat even a tiny bit on fat. REMEMBER THAT!

3. The real news pertains to carbohydrate. Until recently, we thought that while the body may not be quite as efficient at converting excess carbohydrate to body fat as it is in converting dietary fat to body fat, any extra calories still ended up in your fat storage. *We now know that this is not true. Except under very, very unusual circumstances, the body converts almost no carbohydrate to fat!*

THE T-FACTOR CARBOHYDRATE STORY

A bit of history first. We have known for some time that it takes more energy to convert carbohydrate to fat than dietary fat to body fat. The cost of converting dietary fat to body fat is only 3 per cent, which means that only 3 out of every 100 calories of dietary fat will be burned as the body converts fat for storage. In comparison, the cost of going through the various steps that convert carbohydrate to fat is about 25 per cent. That is, whenever the body converts carbohydrate to fat, it takes about 25 per cent of the energy content of the carbohydrate to fuel the conversion process. This leaves about 75 per cent available for fat storage.

Based on these costs as determined in the laboratory, we used to think that should you consume more energy than you expended in a given day, part of it in carbohydrate and part in fat, 97 per cent of the fat and 75 per cent of the carbohydrate ended up in your fat cells.

NOT SO!

Within a very wide range, which I'll discuss below, the body finds a way to burn off or enter into temporary glycogen* storage just about every single bit of the carbohydrate you give it, while only the fat goes to fat. Under normal circumstances, in any given day *a maximum of only about 4 per cent of the carbohydrate is converted to fat*.

Here are some other facts which I hope will convince you of the weight-management value of cutting fat in your diet and substituting carbohydrate.

The body expends from two to three times more energy metabolizing carbohydrate compared with fat. By this I mean it burns two to three times more calories just getting carbohydrates from your intestines into your bloodstream and transforming it to glycogen for storage in your liver and muscles (and eight times more calories to convert any part of it to fat).

If you customarily eat a high-carbohydrate diet, your metabolic rate over a twenty-four-hour period is likely to be higher than the metabolic rate of a person eating a high-fat diet. Although you are not consciously aware of it, a high ratio of carbohydrate to fat in your diet causes your body to work a bit harder after every meal than a high ratio of fat to carbohydrate. This thermic effect of a high-carbohydrate diet can average as much as 200 or even 300 calories each day. These calories are simply burned off and wasted.

In addition, should you ever go out on the town and celebrate with a big meal, your metabolic rate will go even higher in an effort to burn off the extra calories if you normally eat a high-carbohydrate diet rather than a high-fat diet.

Even if you take in a large amount of carbohydrate, practically none of it will be turned to fat. In fact, in one of the studies I describe and reference in Appendix A, the research subjects ate a single meal containing 2000 carbohydrate calories. Only 81 of those calories were turned to fat and, because the body burns a mixture of fat and carbohydrate for fuel, the subjects had to burn stored body fat in the hours that followed that meal. In other words, in spite of consuming 2000 carbohydrate calories in a single sitting, they began to lose body fat!

This sounds so unbelievable that I'm sure you want to know whether there are any conditions at all under which the body will

---

* Glycogen is a polysaccharide, a different form of the carbohydrate that your body stores so that it can be retrieved easily and quickly when needed. After retrieval it is transformed to glucose before being burned as fuel.

begin to convert carbohydrate to fat. The answer is yes, but the conditions are so extreme that I don't think you or anyone else would want to create them intentionally. Here's why.

Because the body seems to resist converting carbohydrate to fat, you must force it to do so. You would have to overeat your daily energy needs for carbohydrate by hundreds or even thousands of calories every day for many successive days to do this. The first few hundred carbohydrate calories of your overconsumption will be fitted into your liver and muscle storage sites. But these sites fill rather quickly. Then, in an effort to burn off any additional carbohydrate, your body gradually increases its metabolic rate. To maintain the conversion of carbohydrate to fat, you would have to keep on increasing your food consumption, eating more and more carbohydrate every day. Overeating in this way is not at all like overeating at a single meal. Most of us would not voluntarily wish to endure the experience! I discuss the research that demonstrates this in Appendix A.

HOW THE BODY STORES FUEL

Carbohydrate is transformed into glucose, a form of sugar that your body can use directly as fuel. But then, since we only use a part of the carbohydrate we eat at any given meal immediately, most of it is transformed to another form of sugar, called glycogen, for storage. Your body has limited room for glycogen storage: About 400 calories are normally stored in the liver plus 1200 to 1600 calories in muscle tissue. That amount can be increased by a few hundred calories through exercise, which encourages your muscles to store some extra energy, or, as I described above, by greatly overeating on carbohydrate, which saturates all storage sites.

The glycogen is stored in a solution of water, about 3 to 4 parts water to 1 part glycogen. For every 500 calories of glycogen stored enough water is combined with it to equal 1 pound of body weight. Thus, whenever you increase or decrease just 500 calories of your glycogen stores, you gain or lose a pound of body weight, but it's mostly water. Part of the daily weight fluctuation we all experience is due to variation in our carbohydrate intake, as well as our salt intake, which also influences water retention.

Quick-weight-loss diets that cut out carbohydrates in the diet capitalise on glycogen depletion to give you a spurious weight loss; the water weight is regained immediately upon any increase in calorie consumption.

Fat, in contrast with glycogen, can be stored in almost unlimited quantities. A woman of normal weight may have 85,000 to 100,000 calories in fat storage, and with a high-fat diet and a lack of physical activity, fat storage is easily increased. A person who is 2 stone (13 kg) overweight has about 105,000 extra calories in fat storage, on top of the average of 85,000 to 100,000 in someone of normal weight.

Fat is stored in a ratio of 4 parts fat to 1 part water. This is almost the exact *opposite* ratio of carbohydrate to water. And because there are 9 calories contained in each gram of fat, compared with only 4 in each gram of glycogen, this means that each pound of fat contains about 3500 calories. Do you see what this energy concentration in fat storage implies for weight loss? While you will lose a pound of mostly water for every 500-calorie deficit in carbohydrate intake, it takes a deficit of 3500 calories to lose a pound of fat. But don't jump to conclusions! When you cut back on calories, you deplete glycogen stores quickly and lose a lot of water weight, but since you have only about 2000 calories in your glycogen stores, this rate of loss is severely limited. It cannot last.

Fast-weight-loss diets that cut back on carbohydrates count on the water loss that accompanies the depletion of your glycogen stores to make the diets more attractive and encourage you to try them. They also count on the cutback in sodium (salt) intake that accompanies a reduction in calories, which also leads to a large water loss. But, at the end of one to two weeks, you've reached a new low point in glycogen storage and in water balance. At that time, weight loss, while now all fat,* is about seven times slower than it was when you first began to diet. If you don't understand how the nature of your diet affects water balance and weight loss, this slowdown can be very discouraging.

HOW THE BODY BURNS FUEL

Under normal circumstances your body burns all the protein you can eat in a day. As I described above, the new research shows that, short of 'force feeding', we also burn all the carbohydrate we eat. Since, within a very wide range, we tend to burn in our fuel mix each day all the protein and carbohydrate that we obtain in our diets, the difference between our total daily energy needs and the combined amount of energy that was supplied by protein and carbohydrate must be made up by burning fat.

---

* When people who are greatly overweight lose weight they also lose a certain amount of lean tissue simply because they don't need as much muscle to carry excess weight around. This is perfectly normal.

THE FAT CAN COME FROM OUR DIETS OR OUT OF OUR FAT CELLS!

This is a very important point. It is essential that you understand what it means for weight control. Let me show you how it works with a real example from an important research study.

In this study the research subjects ate two breakfasts, on different days, that had exactly the same amount of protein and carbohydrate, but varied in fat content.

On each of the two days, the diet had 120 calories in protein and 292 calories in carbohydrate.

On the low-fat day it had only 54 calories in fat.

On the high-fat day it contained 414 calories in fat.

After each of the breakfasts, the researchers measured the amounts of protein, carbohydrate, and fat that were burned by these subjects in their fuel mixtures during the next nine hours.

On both days the total energy needs over nine hours were quite similar – the research subjects burned about 760 to 780 calories. On each of the days they burned almost exactly the same number of protein and carbohydrate calories as were contained in the breakfast, that is, about 120 protein calories and about 292 carbohydrate calories. The really interesting results concern fat, because on both days the subjects burned approximately 360 calories of fat in their fuel mixtures.

That is, regardless of the fat content of the breakfast – it didn't matter whether it was high or low – the body still burned the same total calories and the same amount of fat.

But, as you can see illustrated in Figure 2.1, ON THE LOW-FAT DAY, THE BODY TOOK ABOUT 300 CALORIES OUT OF FAT STORAGE. ON THE HIGH-FAT DAY, THE BODY USED THE DIETARY FAT IN ITS FUEL MIXTURE AND HAD ABOUT 50 CALORIES LEFT OVER TO BE PUT INTO FAT STORAGE!

The research I have just discussed, together with the other studies I present in Appendix A, has led us to the amazing conclusion that when it comes to the amount of fat you have in storage – the fat that's making you overweight – the calories that you consume in the form of protein and carbohydrate don't really count for very much. You, as well as everyone else concerned with remedying the problem of obesity, must revise your way of thinking. It's not a question of total calories and you don't have to cut them down and go on low-calorie diets in order to lose weight.

The reason you got fat in the first place is that you took in more calories in the form of dietary fat than you were burning off in your daily fuel mixture.

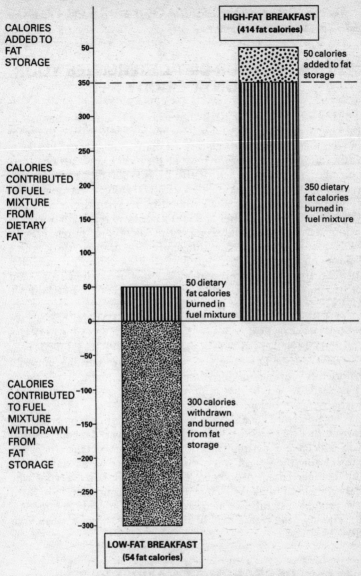

Figure 2-1: Source of fat burned in fuel mixture following low- and high-fat breakfasts. In the nine hours following both breakfasts an average of 350 calories in fat was burned in the fuel mixture. On the low-fat day only about 50 calories in fat was supplied in the diet, thus requiring that about 300 fat calories be withdrawn from fat cells. On the high-fat day approximately 400 calories were contained in the diet. Since the fuel mixture only required about 350 calories there were about 50 calories left over to be added to fat storage (figures are rounded for ease of illustration: see text for details.).

And the key to losing weight, in the simplest of terms, is to eat less fat in your daily diet than your body burns each day.

THE FAT IN YOUR DIET DETERMINES YOUR AMOUNT OF BODY FAT

The research I have discussed above has led leading biochemists to the conclusion that body fat may be more closely related to the fat in your diet than to total calories. As in the study described above, within a wide range, you will burn up the protein and carbohydrate you need each day. Then, if the fat in your diet exceeds your remaining needs for energy, it goes into fat storage. As long as you continue to eat more fat than you burn in your fuel mix each day you will keep getting fatter and fatter until you reach a new equilibrium where the expanded energy needs of your fatter, heavier body match your high fat intake. In one animal study where calories and the mixture of nutrients could be controlled carefully, an increase from 20 per cent of calories in fat to 40 per cent of calories in fat led to A DOUBLING OF BODY-FAT CONTENT.

THEREFORE, THE KEY TO A PERMANENT LOW AMOUNT OF BODY FAT IS NOT CUTTING CALORIES OR 'DIETING'. IT'S A PERMANENT LOW-FAT DIET.

The T-Factor Diet makes sure that you are burning more fat calories in your fuel mixture than you are consuming in your diet. This leads to weight loss of *fat* even if you increase your carbohydrate consumption.

The T-Factor Diet also shows you how to maintain a permanent low-fat diet that you can like and enjoy for ever. This means that you will have a permanently lower body-fat content when you finish losing the weight you want to lose. Since we all start with a different percentage of body fat, I can't promise that everyone who halves their fat intake will cut their body-fat content in half. But I can promise a significant, permanent reduction, and the more you have to lose, the greater will be the impact of reducing fat in your diet.

RESEARCH AT VANDERBILT

What, in actual practice, occurs when you use the T-Factor Diet? Can we determine the amount of body fat you are likely to burn off each day? How much weight will you lose and how fast?

RESEARCH IN THE CALORIMETRY CHAMBER

In one phase of our studies, research subjects live for twenty-four-hour periods in a calorimetry chamber. This room, which is like a small motel room with all amenities, contains a TV, video, telephone and exercise equipment, together with other facilities, such as a commode, basin and small refrigerator. It is also airtight. Since we supply the air to the room, we can measure the change in the expired gas as the subjects breathe throughout the day and night. The room is also equipped with radar and we can monitor the amount of physical activity that occurs spontaneously. This provides us with a means of determining with great accuracy the daily metabolic rate, the response to different diets and exercise levels, and the proportions of fat and carbohydrate that are burned each day in the fuel mixture.

Subjects in our research are acclimatized to living on two separate diets, a high-fat, low-carbohydrate diet or a low-fat, high-carbohydrate diet (T-Factor fat-gram intake), for a full week at a time. We measure the daily energy needs and the nature of the fuel mixture during two separate days of each of these weeks during which they spend twenty-four hours in the chamber. We then repeat the process again with the same subject in order to verify and replicate the findings of the first two weeks.

We have determined that the thermic effect of food – that's the amount of energy it takes to metabolize food over and above the resting metabolic rate – can average as much as 200 calories or more on a high-carbohydrate diet each day compared with as little as 50 calories on a high-fat diet *in the same individual*. That's energy that is not available for sustaining metabolic functions or for storage. It's wasted.

In addition, when the same individual switches to the low-fat T-Factor Diet, the fuel mixture still requires considerably more fat than is contained in the diet. During the week on the T-Factor Diet, an average of over 100 calories more each day is withdrawn from the fat cells, compared with a high-fat diet for the same subject.

Obviously, the greater thermic response to the high-carbohydrate diet and the need for more fat in the fuel mixture than is contained in the diet can lead to weight loss. This helps explain the fine results we have obtained with the T-Factor Diet in our clinical studies.

CLINICAL STUDIES AT VANDERBILT

In our clinical studies with two different groups of women, we contrasted the weight loss and reactions to the T-Factor Diet in its two forms, the basic, no calorie counting or cutting form, and the Quick Melt.

The Quick Melt is calorie controlled around a core menu of about 1000 calories per day. A snack is permitted (in fact, recommended so that subjects will not feel deprived and can maintain the diet for as long as they choose). As implemented by our research subjects in actual practice, the Quick Melt ended up at about 1250 calories per day. Subjects in the no counting or cutting group ended up eating about 1500 calories a day. For identification purposes in our study, we called this latter group the Lifestyle group.

Both groups followed the T-Factor fat gram formula and, over time, both groups averaged approximately 30 grams of fat per day, or about 270 calories. The extra 250 calories eaten by the Lifestyle group were almost entirely in the form of carbohydrate snacks. All subjects were encouraged to gradually increase physical activity until they could walk comfortably at a brisk pace for 45 minutes.

The average amount overweight according to standard weight for height tables in our groups was just over 4 stone (27 kg), and the average age of the women was thirty-nine. Just about all were quite sedentary before beginning this programme.

As you might expect, the Quick Melt group lost weight rapidly, averaging 11 pounds (5 kg) in the first three weeks, and then slowing to an average of between 1.5 and 2 pounds (700–900 g) per week thereafter. The Lifestyle group lost an average of 7 pounds (3 kg) in the first three weeks, and then slowed to about 1 pound (450 g) a week thereafter. Several of the women in the Lifestyle group lost over a stone (7 kg) during the first five weeks. This was a great surprise to me. I never anticipated that our research subjects would achieve that speed of loss without making a conscious effort to curtail eating and cut calories. Of course, by reducing fat they did end up eating fewer calories than before, *but they also ate far more food in terms of bulk and weight than ever before. They were never hungry.* Needless to say, our research subjects were very pleased. In Chapter Four I will reproduce some of their personal reactions, as well as my own and those of the Vanderbilt Weight Management Program's director of nutrition as we adopted the T-Factor Diet.

A FIELD STUDY

There is always a problem in extrapolating from a controlled study, in which seriously overweight research subjects are guided and monitored by a professional staff, to what might happen to that great mass of people 'in the real world' who only want to lose a small amount of weight. What can we expect when people adopt the T-Factor fat gram formula on their own and follow the general recommendations that I give to you in Chapter Three?

Although not planned as a formal study, after two lectures on nutrition and obesity given by Ms Pope-Cordle and me, eight young women and one man between the ages of 19 and 22 decided to count fat grams and follow the T-Factor formula for a minimum of two weeks as part of their project that term in a Health Promotion Course at Vanderbilt University. The women were all within the normal weight range, with weights lying between the mid and upper points of the suggested weight table. The man was 8 pounds (3.5 kg) above the upper limit. Thus, these women (and the man) were all concerned with what has been called 'the final 5 to 15' pounds that millions of people, but especially women, struggle with all their lives and never seem to be rid of once and for all.

The women averaged a loss of 1.25 pounds (560 g) per week during the project. Out of curiosity alone, since this was not a research study, I decided to survey the group without prior warning at the end of the semester. You can imagine how pleased I was to discover that they had ALL stuck with the T-Factor Diet and that they had averaged, *and maintained*, exactly the loss they set out for: 5 pounds (2.25 kg). The man lost 11 pounds (5 kg) in one month, and he, too, had maintained that loss at follow-up. EVERY SINGLE PERSON WAS SUCCESSFUL.

It is important in considering these results to note that the people who achieved them did so without participating in a formal research study. Thus they had no external motivation or supervision supplied by a group leader, and there was no external motivation to continue with the programme in anticipation of a follow-up.

Why – indeed, HOW – had all of these students continued to stick with the T-Factor Diet? If you have ever tried to eat a healthy diet as a student living on campus, you will know what I mean when I emphasise that word 'how'. Well, as one of the young women remarked in the comments section of her follow-up form, 'It's easy and it works!'

CHAPTER THREE

PUTTING THE T-FACTOR DIET TO WORK: HOW TO LOSE WEIGHT WITHOUT CUTTING CALORIES

It's not how much you eat, but WHAT you eat.

If you've ever been on a diet I'm sure you remember the *energy equation* the experts refer to when they suggest that you cut back on your calorie intake to lose weight. This equation states that you maintain your weight when

$$\text{ENERGY IN} = \text{ENERGY OUT}$$

Then, in order to lose weight, you are told to 'unbalance the energy equation.' *Energy in* must be less than *energy out*.

Energy in is considered to be the energy content of the food in your diet, as measured in the laboratory. These are the calories listed in your calorie counters. In the previous chapter I explained that this is not an entirely correct way to view energy balance when it comes to weight management. The energy that is available for use or that gets stored in the human body from protein and carbohydrate IS NOT EQUAL when compared with fat. And, similarly, all *energy out* is also not equal when it comes to losing body fat, but I'll discuss this issue when I deal with physical activity in Chapter Eight.

The key to losing excess body fat is not simply a question of relating the total energy in your diet to your total energy expenditure. Changes in body fat depend primarily on that portion of the energy in or out that is supplied by fat. If you eat less fat each day than the fat you are burning up in the fuel mixture required to sustain your basal metabolic processes and the fat you are using to power physical activity, you end up losing body fat. In other words, when

$$\text{FAT } IN \text{ is less than FAT } OUT$$

you will lose weight, and 100 per cent of the weight you lose will be FAT.

22

I must emphasise this fact – the way to lose body fat is to eat less fat than you burn up each day.

Of course you can rush the process and cut back on calories, too, if you want to lose weight even more quickly. This will pull calories out of both your carbohydrate and fat stores, and I'll discuss the best way to do this when I talk about the Quick Melt in Chapter Five. But when you follow the T-Factor Diet as I will outline in this chapter, we are concerned only with the fat in your diet, not cutting calories.

DO YOU KNOW HOW MUCH FAT IS CONTAINED IN THE FOOD YOU EAT EACH DAY?

I'll bet you don't! Our research shows that the great majority of people do not know how much fat they eat each day. Even those of us who are most nutrition and weight conscious think 'calories', not 'fat'. We know that butter, ice cream, chips and mayonnaise are fatty foods, but we don't realize that 50 to 75 per cent of calories in many meat and dairy products, snack foods, dressings and puddings are fat calories.

Once you know where the fat in your diet is coming from and become aware of how much you consume each day, it's not hard to make some modifications and design a satisfying diet that will start melting off *all* your surplus body fat. Follow the general principles that I will outline in this chapter. Within a matter of weeks I think you will find that you are able to modify your present diet and develop a new approach to eating that will become the most satisfying régime that you've ever enjoyed. You will never feel hungry because you can add anything you want to the basic diet so long as it isn't a fatty food. And, as a bonus, if you have been eating a typical Western diet and suffering from any kind of gastric distress, you will probably feel better than you have ever felt before.

FORGET ABOUT CALORIES!

The first thing you need to do when you follow the T-Factor Diet without cutting calories is to forget about them! When you follow the T-Factor Diet you need make no effort to count calories. Don't even think calories. This way you never feel that you are 'dieting'. We are only going to make some substitutions.

You will be amazed at the freedom from food obsessions that this will give you. Rather than feeling guilty about every deviation from a calorie goal, you will be quite happy about the easy switches from high- to low-fat foods that will soon become habitual.

But there is still some work to do. At first you will need to count fat grams, so you are not entirely free from counting. You must learn where the fat in your diet is coming from, and we are con-

23

cerned with grams of fat. I'll explain how we do this in a moment when I give you our 'magic'* formula for losing fat without dieting.

Counting grams of fat, however, lasts only until you learn the fat content of the differing foods and recipes that will become part of your customary diet. The major difference between the T-Factor Diet and other diets is that you don't have to restrain yourself to fit within some calorie limit. Our only concern is with fat. You are free to make healthy substitutions for fatty foods *and to keep on eating healthy foods until your appetite is satisfied*. No more guilt feelings!

Strangely enough, an interesting issue arose when the T-Factor Diet was first introduced to our research participants at Vanderbilt. I was greeted by a roomful of sceptical faces. They couldn't believe that they could lose weight simply by exchanging nutrients—carbohydrate for fat—and still eat pretty much to their heart's content. Well, as the saying goes, the proof of the pudding is in the eating.

I will describe my own experience when I switched to the T-Factor Diet, and those of some other individuals, in Chapter Four. According to the weight charts, I did not need to lose weight. I was right in the middle of the desirable weight range. But I certainly did not want to talk about this fascinating new dietary concept without living it out myself. I lost 7 pounds (3 kg) in seven weeks simply by changing the composition of my diet, and all of it from the nice little extra store of fat around my hips! The others whom I interviewed had lost as much as 3½ stone (23 kg) or more. The T-Factor Diet has led to some remarkable changes in our lives, and together we'll give you some useful tips.

THE 'MAGIC' NUMBERS

I've been talking about grams, not calories, and it's grams of fat that we are concerned with in the T-Factor Diet. Perhaps some of you have counted carbohydrate grams as part of a weight-control effort in the past, thinking that it was carbohydrates that were

---

* My colleagues and I debated the use of the word 'magic', which I have put in quotation marks, because we don't want to be misunderstood. There is no magical cure for obesity. Permanent changes in diet and/or activity level are necessary to achieve a permanent change in weight. I made a decision to keep the word, in quotation marks, to communicate an 'as if' quality. The T-Factor concept is so simple to implement, compared to calorie counting and cutting, that the results may truly seem unbelievable, if not 'magical', to you.

responsible for your weight problems. We now know that it's the fat that counts, almost to the exclusion of other forms of energy.

A gram of fat contains approximately 9 calories, compared with approximately 4 contained in a gram of carbohydrate. You will soon get a feeling for where the fat lies in the foods you customarily eat. The menus in this chapter all contain fat-gram counts and there are a number of discussions below that will alert you to the differences in foods as you begin to make low-fat for high-fat substitutions. You will, of course, study the Fat and Fibre Counter in Appendix C.

Our studies show that the average overweight woman is eating between 80 and 100 grams of fat each day. That, translated into calories, is between 720 and 900 calories in fat. The average man is taking in about 20 grams more, or between 900 and 1080 calories in fat.

The T-Factor formula for weight loss is:

20 to 40 grams of fat per day for women
30 to 60 grams of fat per day for men

Men can eat more fat than women and still lose weight because they have higher energy needs. The range is large to allow for flexibility. Even at 40 grams a day, most women will be cutting their fat intake in half, and will lose weight, although not as fast as they would if they chose to stay near the bottom of the range.

Only fat grams are limited. When you have reached your quota of fat grams for the day, you may substitute no-fat foods for foods with fat at any time until your appetite is satisfied. I'll give more details on how to implement this formula as we go along.

It's not wise to go below the ranges that I suggest because fat supplies some essential nutrients that cannot be obtained from other foods and a minimal amount is necessary for the transport of fat-soluble vitamins. Besides, fat makes food taste good. If you don't get enough fat, you are likely to feel deprived. *Deprived people are more likely to binge.* Do not deprive yourself. The T-Factor Diet is to be enjoyed. It's not a penance.

With respect to protein, the T-Factor Diet recommends levels and types of protein foods that are common in the Western world, although I will be showing you healthy and tasty ways to switch a portion of your animal protein intake to vegetable sources. So, assuming an adequate protein intake, you are, as I've indicated, free to compensate for the reduction of fat in your diet with whatever increase in carbohydrate foods satisfies your appetite.

Because of the greater weight and volume of carbohydrate foods, compared with fatty foods, you will probably cut back a bit in calories, too. This automatic cut is another benefit that accrues from the T-Factor Diet without conscious effort, and it serves to foster a speedier loss of weight.

Since you don't have to cut fat to unreasonable levels, food still tastes good. You obtain yet another big plus because the nutritional value of your diet will improve immensely. Calorie for calorie, carbohydrate foods, especially the complex carbohydrates in fruits, vegetables, and whole grains, have far more vitamins and minerals than fatty foods.

FIRST STEPS FIRST

I realize, of course, that you probably are not accustomed to thinking in terms of fat grams rather than calories. So, when you first start to implement the T-Factor Diet you will need to do several things to make it easy for yourself.

1. As you read this chapter, be sure to study carefully the list of foods in Table 3.1 and plan how you will make the suggested low-fat substitutions for any high-fat foods in your present diet. A study of that table will give you a feeling for food fat content in general, high versus low, and start you thinking about how you will make substitutions.

2. Study my discussions on food preparation and menu design below. These will provide you with your first steps towards gaining more specific information on the fat-gram content of different foods.

I will present you with some specific suggestions for a selection of 'standard' breakfasts and lunches (all with fat-gram content of the suggested foods). Most people eat about three different kinds of breakfasts and, similarly, a rather restricted number of different lunches. I want you to think in terms of several kinds of breakfasts and lunches that you can live with just as comfortably as your present selection. If you don't care for my specific suggests, you will be able to design your own using the Fat and Fibre Counter in Appendix C. You can use my suggestions as models. Not that you will be unable to deviate occasionally and have an old-fashioned traditional breakfast. Of course you will. Preferably before doing a day of old-fashioned physical activity! But the standard low-fat breakfasts and lunches will ensure that you fall within the fat-gram limits on most days.

3. I also present suggestions for five standard dinners that you can include in your diet whenever the spirit moves you. Each includes a different, easily prepared main course that is attractive and interesting. My recipes will show you how to select and prepare

26

these dishes, which most of us already include in our diets, but from now on with a minimum of fat.

However, for a full introduction to the great variety and gastronomic pleasure offered in the T-Factor Diet, I encourage you to try the entire twenty-one days of menus that I present as models in this chapter (pages 42–52). My colleagues and I have designed these menus to take you through a large range of different foods and styles of cooking. In a way, we intend these menus to furnish a practical education in nutrition. Represented in these menus you will find just about everything available in your local supermarket. All common fruits, vegetables, low-fat meats, and so on. We have recipes to help you learn how to prepare these foods in a healthy way. AND IF YOU THINK HEALTHY, LOW-FAT COOKING IS A BORE AND A BOTHER, I WANT YOU TO TRY EVERY SINGLE ONE OF THE VEGETABLE, GRAIN, AND MEATLESS MAIN COURSE RECIPES. Let us show you the way to increase your culinary repertoire and help everyone around you to stay slim and healthier.

You will notice that our menus specify portion sizes only for foods that contain more than trace amounts of fat; other foods are unlimited, although you can adjust your intake to promote whatever speed of weight loss you prefer.

4. Until you have a good idea of how to construct a diet that falls within the 20- to 40-gram fat limit for women or the 30- to 60-gram range for men, you must count fat grams every day. Before you begin the T-Factor Diet, it is a good idea to skim through the more complete list in the Fat and Fibre Counter in Appendix C, which gives fat grams per serving of many common foods. You need to know where the fat grams are and this list will give you a broad guide to food selection, especially when you desire to make substitutions for anything in the menus. NOTE THAT SOME FOODS HAVE SO LITTLE FAT THAT THEY CAN BE EATEN IN UNLIMITED QUANTITIES AT ANY TIME, AS PART OF YOUR MEALS OR AS UNLIMITED SNACKS.

WHY THE EMPHASIS ON FIBRE IN THE T-FACTOR DIET, AND WHICH FATS ARE BEST?

Before giving you specific instructions for the T-Factor Diet I must make a digression and talk about the health benefits of increasing fibre in your diet and the reasons for replacing some of the animal fat with fats from vegetables, nuts or seeds.

I am sure you are aware of the efforts that are being made by health professionals to get us to increase our fibre intake. Certain forms of fibre, such as the non-soluble kinds found in whole-grain wheat and wheat bran, seem to help to reduce the likelihood of intestinal cancer. Others, such as the water-soluble kinds contained in whole oats and oat bran, rice bran, many fruits, peas, legumes, and sweetcorn, seem to help reduce cholesterol and thus the likelihood of cardiovascular disease. Almost every month another article is published in some medical or nutrition journal that reports health benefits for one or another of the high-fibre foods. Similarly, just about as frequently you will find another article reporting the dangers of high-fat consumption, especially of saturated fats, which are found primarily in products of animal origin or in palm or coconut oil. While there is evidence that fibre may help counteract to some slight extent the effects of too much fat in the diet by binding with it and preventing some of it from being absorbed, most of us would do well to attack the problem directly and reduce fat in general.

Although a reduction in total fat should be your primary consideration, you may obtain additional health benefits by replacing a good part of the animal fats in your diet with mono-unsaturated and poly-unsaturated fats. Fats of animal origin are highly saturated and encourage the body to increase its production of cholesterol. Some experts believe saturated fat is an even greater danger in its ability to foster cholesterol production than is dietary cholesterol itself, partly because we tend to consume so much of it. Saturated fats tend to be solid at room temperature. Except for palm and coconut oil, which are also highly saturated, fats from vegetables, nuts, and seeds are mono- and poly-unsaturated, and liquid at room temperature. Soft margarines tend to be less saturated than hard margarines. I use primarily the mono-unsaturated oils, such as olive oil for my salads and groundnut oil for cooking. The flavour of olive oil makes it the best for salad dressings, while groundnut oil withstands higher temperatures. Research reports suggest that consumption of both these oils, as well as other mono-unsaturated oils, can lower your cholesterol level.

By reducing saturated fat, switching to the use of mono- and poly-unsaturated fats, and increasing soluble fibre in the diet, you may achieve a significant reduction in cholesterol level. Reductions of 20 per cent or more are common, and the process is accentuated when you lose weight.

But the role of fibre in the T-Factor Diet is important for many other reasons. Fibre is most commonly found in exactly the foods you can eat in virtually unlimited quantities without gaining weight. When you reduce the fat in your diet, it is next to impossible to eat enough of these foods – the complex carbohydrates – to interfere with gradual weight loss.

The goal for fibre is 20 to 40 grams a day for a woman, and as high as 50 grams for a man. Many people find they can eat even more than that without any ill effects.

However, don't go wild over fibre and immediately make a drastic increase. If you have been eating a typical Western low-fibre diet (10 to 12 grams a day), YOU MUST INCREASE GRADUALLY. If you triple your intake overnight you may suffer some intestinal distress, including wind, possibly diarrhoea, or even constipation if you don't drink enough liquid. The digestive system can adapt, at least partially if not completely, to an increase in fibre *over time*. So any distress you notice is likely to disappear as your body adjusts to a change in diet.

While fibre can prevent the absorption of about 10 per cent of the fat you eat each day, certain forms of fibre in very large quantities can also interfere with the absorption of certain vitamins and minerals. This is a very complex subject and details are not relevant to the T-Factor Diet. I want to be sure you understand, however, that there is no danger of harmful absorption interference with the T-Factor Diet. The recommended fibre intake is within the safe range and, because you end up eating so many healthy foods as you reduce your fat intake, the 'nutrient density' of your diet increases dramatically. That is, when fat goes down in the diet and whole grains, fruits, and vegetables increase, the amount of vitamins and minerals in the diet per 1000 calories is significantly increased.

The key to getting enough of the several different kinds of healthy fibre is to eat a wide variety of foods. Once again, there is no need to become obsessed with getting enough of each kind. You will find the variety you need in my menus and recipes, where I make use of different grains in breads, muffins and side dishes, often combined with legumes. Of course, there's plenty of fruit and vegetables. So long as you eat a wide variety of foods, there is no need to become obsessed about *anything* in your diet. And that goes for fat and fibre, too. Once you see where the fat and fibre lie, eating healthy foods will become a matter of habit and you won't need to count grams of fat and fibre any more, just as there is no need to count calories.

CUTTING BACK ON FATS

The T-Factor Diet does not require you to cut out any particular group of foods in order to meet the fat-gram goal of 20 to 40, or 30 to 60, grams a day. I will show you how to use butter, oil and other fats in moderation. But there is also a large amount of hidden fat in many cuts of meat, dairy products, seafood prepared in rich sauces, sweets, and snack foods. Since we want to keep low-fat versions of these foods in the diet, you will want to learn how to make low-fat substitutions for the high-fat foods in the same food group.

On the right-hand side of Table 3.1 you will find a list of high-fat foods commonly found in the diets of fat people. On the left-hand side are good low-fat substitutions. This table contains my general suggestions for making a real dent in your fat intake. It's intended to give a gut feeling for where the fat lies in your diet. We will get into fat-gram specifics in a moment.

Looking at Table 3.1, do you see how you can keep on eating all kinds of meat and dairy products and certain snacks and desserts and still make a great dent in your fat intake? By making good choices it is very easy to cut out half the fat in most diets without causing any feeling of deprivation at all.

Table 3.2 contains a list of grains, fruits, and vegetables that contain no more than a trace of fat – that is, less than 0.5 gram in the case of the fruits and vegetables, and less than 1 gram in the grains. There is generally a small amount of fat in a whole-grain food, which is contained in the germ or husk. That's why even dry cereal products made without added fat but which contain whole grains usually list a small amount per serving. Watch out for certain cereals, however, which contain considerable added fat in spite of their healthy-sounding names. Read the labels.

TABLE 3.1
FAT SUBSTITUTION GUIDE

USE	INSTEAD OF
Skimmed or low-fat milk	Whole milk or cream
Evaporated skimmed milk (tinned)	Cream, whipping cream
Plain low-fat or skimmed-milk yoghurt	Sour cream
Low-fat cottage cheese (sieved or whizzed)	Cream cheese or sour cream
Low-fat cheeses	High-fat cheeses
½ tin soup and ½ tin skimmed milk	Whole tin of cream soup (in recipes)
Sorbet, low-fat desserts	Ice cream
Low-fat yoghurt with fresh fruit	Commercial yoghurts with fruit, sugar
2 egg whites	One whole egg (in recipes)
Reduced-calorie mayonnaise, mustard, ketchup	Ordinary mayonnaise

TABLE 3.1 *cont.*

No-cal or low-cal salad dressings	Ordinary salad dressings
½ or less of the fat called for in recipes, topped up with a suitable liquid	Ordinary amount of fat (in recipes)
Blend of yoghurt and mayonnaise	Salad dressing for tuna, chicken
Lean, well-trimmed meats, under 15% fat (flank, fillet or topside)	Heavily marbelled cuts, over 15% fat
Minced turkey	Minced beef
Chicken, turkey without skin	Poultry with skin, duck
Water-(brine-) packed fish	Fish tinned in oil
Fresh fish, grilled, baked, poached, steamed	Fried fish, frozen breaded fish
Measured portions of meat Women: up to 7 oz/200 g per day Men: up to 9 oz/250 g per day	Large portions of meat
Low-fat sauces and marinades	High-fat sauces and gravies
Bouillon, herbs, wine, juices	Gravy, fatty sauces
Low-fat cooking methods: grill, bake, boil, poach, steam	High-fat cooking methods: fry, cook in own fat
Legumes, beans, peas, tofu	Meats
Meatless sauces	Sauces containing meat
Steamed or microwaved vegetables seasoned with herbs, spices, lemon juice, low-fat sauces	Vegetables in margarine/ butter or cheese sauce, or fried vegetables
Water chestnuts	Nuts in vegetable casseroles
Unsweetened water- or juice-packed tinned or frozen fruits	Sweetened or syrup-packed tinned or frozen fruits
Fresh or dried fruits	High-fat snacks, biscuits or puddings
Fresh fruit with juice or cottage cheese	Butter or syrup, sugar or cream on pancakes, biscuits or cakes

TABLE 3.1 *cont.*

Water, soda or mineral water, tea, coffee	Milkshakes
Pretzels	Crisps, nuts
Raw vegetables, low-fat dips	Crisps, nuts, packeted snacks
Low-fat yoghurt or tofu dips	Sour-cream dips
Whole-grain bread, oatcakes, rice cakes, low-fat cripsbreads	Doughnuts, biscuits, cakes
Mashed potato topping	Pastry
Angel food cake	Higher-fat cakes
Fresh fruit	Higher-fat desserts
Puddings made with skimmed milk	Puddings made with whole milk
Jelly or jam on toast or bread	Butter or margarine on toast or bread

TABLE 3.2
FRUIT, VEGETABLES, AND GRAIN FOODS HAVING LITTLE OR NO FAT*
(you do not need to control your consumption of these foods)

FRUIT
(fresh)

Apple	Mango	Pineapple
Banana	Melon	Plum
Blackberries	Orange	Raspberries
Cherries	Papaya	Rhubarb
Grapefruit	Peach	Strawberries
Grapes	Pear	Tangerine
Kiwi	Persimmon	Watermelon

(dried)

Apple	Papaya	Prunes
Apricot	Peach	Raisins
Dates	Pear	Sultanas
Figs	Pineapple	

VEGETABLES

Asparagus	Beetroot	Cabbage
Aubergine	Broccoli	Carrots
Beansprouts	Brussels sprouts	Cauliflower

TABLE 3.2 *cont.*

Celery	Green pepper	Radishes
Chard	Kale	Runner beans
Chicory	Lettuce	Spinach
Courgettes	Mushrooms	Spring greens
Cucumbers	Mustard and cress	Summer squash
Dandelion greens	Okra	Swede
Endive	Onions	Tomatoes
Escarole	Parsley	Turnips
French beans	Pumpkin	Watercress

GRAINS, LEGUMES, AND OTHER STARCHY FOODS
BREADS

Baps	Pitta bread	Rusks
Bread	Rice cakes	Tortilla
Melba toast	Rolls	

BREAKFAST CEREALS

Many cold and hot breakfast cereals contain no fat to 1 gram of fat per serving. Check the labels of your favourite brands

CRISPBREADS

Bread sticks	Rice cakes	Saltines
Oyster crackers	Ryvita	Water biscuits
Pretzels		

GRAINS AND GRAIN FOODS

Macaroni	Rice	Sweetcorn
Noodles	Spaghetti	Wheat (bulghur, etc.)

LEGUMES AND OTHER STARCHY FOODS

Broad beans	Lentils	Red beans
Chick peas	Peas	Runner beans
Dried beans	Potatoes	Sweet potatoes
French beans		

---

* Fruit and vegetables that contain only trace amounts (less than 0.5 gram) of fat per serving. The grain and other starchy foods usually have less than 1 gram of fat per serving. Be sure to check the labels on all commercially prepared foods for added fat.

ADDITIONAL HINTS FOR CUTTING FATS

Here are some more specific hints for cutting fats. In part, these explain and amplify some of the suggestions in Table 3.1 and I expand on them here because they constitute my personal strategies for controlling fat intake. They work!

1. If you are eating more beef, lamb or pork than poultry or fish, reverse that ratio. And when you do eat beef, lamb, or pork, use the leanest cuts and trim away all fat. The Fat and Fibre Counter will inform you of the relative fat content of various cuts, but, best of all, make friends with your butcher. I really like my butcher. Sometimes exactly what I want is prepackaged on the shelf at the supermarket; when I can't see it there I tell the butcher what I want and he cuts it specially for me. Use my recipes to discover that low-fat substitutions and low-fat food preparation can be even more satisfying than your present way.

2. *Don't eat fried foods. Full stop.* Frying can turn a wonderfully healthy food into a junk food. For example, a potato contains no fat, but turn even a little one into just a small helping of chips and you end up with about 24 grams of fat. That's about 200 calories of fat that could come out of your fat cells instead of going in. It's even worse when you fry chicken or fish coated with breadcrumbs or batter. So when it comes to these foods, bake, grill, steam, poach or occasionally stew or barbecue instead of frying.

3. Cultivate your taste for meatless meals, or try dishes in which the animal products are used for flavouring, as in Oriental cooking. This is one of the easiest ways to cut down on fats. Because Oriental and similar styles of cooking are less familiar and most people think it's a bother to cook this way, try my recipes to get the hang of it.

4. Switch from whole milk to either low-fat or skimmed milk. Use low-fat cottage cheese and yoghurt, and low-fat cheeses whenever possible. You may like the low-fat processed cheese foods, and if you do, I have no objection to them. I don't care for them, however, and prefer to use the best-tasting cheeses more moderately rather than the less satisfying, reduced-fat varieties.

5. Substitute fruit (including dried fruit) for most of your desserts and snacks.

6. Do not use gravies and sauces made with more than minimal amounts of butter and cream. See my low-fat recipes for instruction as to how to use just enough of the fatty ingredients to keep you satisfied.

7. Use all fat and oil in moderation.

But what about diet spreads and commercial calorie-reduced salad dressings? Once again, if you like them, use them. It's a matter of personal choice. We include a couple of recipes that use calorie-reduced products; but, to tell the truth, I don't use most of these products myself. Besides, why pay for water? That's what's often added and homogenized to reduce the fat content while maintaining the weight or volume of the product. When it comes to spreads, or fats like butter and margarine, I think you get more flavour from the real thing even if you use less. As for salad dressings, many people do find a commercial variety that they like, at 35 calories or less per dessertspoonful. That's fine. However, I suggest you try my own recipes for reduced- or no-fat salad dressings. They will illustrate what the best ingredients, including oil used in moderation, can do to satisfy your palate.

HOW TO DEVELOP YOUR DAILY MENU PLAN

Most people alternate between a few standard breakfasts and lunches. I think it's a good idea to include no more than half the fat you plan to eat in a given day in these two meals combined, if you plan to have your main meal at night, as most of us do. Remember, however, that most health experts recommend against eating a large meal before going to sleep. It can interfere with sleep as well as make managing your weight more difficult, and it may be dangerous for people with cardiovascular disease. The size and fat levels of the dinners I recommend are well within good health limits.

Here's an important suggestion. The menus below, as well as my discussion of other foods, contain fat-gram information. Begin to compile your mental storehouse of fat-gram counts. These are the common foods that you will be eating every day. Within a few weeks you will have all the important, everyday fat-gram information in your memory. Choosing low-fat foods will become easy and second nature. You will have to look up fat-gram counts only when you deviate from your customary diet.

BASIC BREAKFASTS

Breakfast in particular can be very low in fat. Here are four of my own standard formulas, plus a yoghurt combination suggested by one of my nutritionist friends. Remember, the only thing you must limit is fat – you can eat the fat-free foods in whatever quantity satisfies you. I include the general, basic fat-gram counts to help you plan your own combinations, but *be sure to check the labels of the brands you use.* There can be considerable differences in the fat content from brand to brand in cereals that have similar names.

Normally we recommend that you drink coffee or tea without milk, but there's room for milk or even a little single cream provided you don't overdo it. Be sure to count it in your fat-gram total.

1

Your choice of fruit or juice
Choice of cereal, cold or hot
(about 1 gram of fat per ounce/28 g cold, or normal helping hot)
Skimmed or low-fat milk
(1 to 2 grams of fat per 4 fl oz/110 ml)
Coffee or tea

2

Choice of fruit or juice
Toast and marmalade
(whole-grain preferred, 1 gram of fat per slice)
Coffee or tea
Add a poached or boiled egg occasionally
(about 5 grams of fat)

3

Choice of fruit
Cheese toast
(9 grams of fat per ounce/28 g of hard cheese,
1 gram of fat per slice of bread)
Coffee or tea

4

Choice of fruit
Choice of muffin
(about 3 grams of fat; see my several muffin recipes)
Coffee or tea

5

Low or very low fat yoghurt mixed with choice of fruit and cold cereal
(1 to 4 grams of fat; check labels of yoghurt and cereal)

When I am really saving fat grams, I may have a couple of slices of hearty whole-grain bread or homemade muffins, plain or toasted, for breakfast. I include two recipes for breads, as well as for American-style muffins made from different grains that are relatively low in fat content and filled with a variety of good fibres. They are great to nibble on at any time.

BASIC LUNCHES
Lunches pose a bit of a problem if you have to eat out every day and

cannot carry your own. While I frequently order salads when I eat out, or soup and salad or a sandwich, I prefer to make my own lunches. The tuna, chicken or ham salads in restaurants will often contain between 12 and 24 grams of fat unless they have been specifically designed as low-fat dishes. If you pour additional dressing on the lettuce and other vegetables that accompany the salad, it's 9 to 10 grams of fat per dessertspoon of the full-fat varieties.

Hearty soups – I mean with potatoes, lentils, rice and plenty of vegetables – are great for lunches. See my recipes; they contain no fat.

Here are some basic fat-gram figures to help you plan your own luncheon combinations. One again, be sure to check the labels of the products you like to use.

1. Tuna fish, packed in water (brine), contains only 1 gram of fat per 3 oz/80 g serving (packed in oil it contains about 20 grams).
2. Low-fat varieties of cottage cheese contain from 2 to 3 grams of fat in each 4 oz/110 g (I know you get tired of seeing cottage cheese and tuna on weight-management menus, so see my suggestions for seasonings on page 153).
3. Bouillon-based soups with added vegetables and potatoes are practically fat-free.
4. Thick vegetable or vegetable, beef and chicken soups will contain about 3 grams of fat per 8 fl oz/225 ml serving (the popular cream soups served in restaurants may contain up to 25 grams of fat).
5. Sardines, oil all drained off, will contain about 6 grams of fat per ½ tin (about 2 oz/56 g).
6. Fruits and vegetables that are virtually fat free (see my lists in Table 3.2 which you can add in unlimited quantities).
7. Bread for sandwiches contains about 1 gram of fat per slice.
8. Mayonnaise is 4 grams per *scant teaspoonful*.
9. Use ketchup and mustard for flavouring.
10. Use lemon juice and vinaigrette dressings, or my own low-fat salad dressings at 4 grams per dessertspoonful.
11. My sandwich spreads (see pages 99–100) contain little or no fat.
12. White meat of chicken or turkey contains about 1 gram of fat per ounce; dark meat contains about 2.5 grams of fat per ounce/28 g.
13. Sliced beef, extra lean, contains about 2.5 grams of fat per ounce/28 g; other cuts about 6 grams per ounce.
14. Ryvita, rice cakes and many other crispbreads have only one or two grams of fat per serving.

With these data in mind, here are some suggestions for lunches that you can repeat over and over again. Note that even the menus with higher fat contents have only about 25 per cent of the day's fat allowance.

1

Choice of soup
(0 to 3 grams of fat)
Water biscuits, Ryvita or toast
(1 to 2 grams of fat per serving)
Unlimited no-fat vegetables and fruits
(see Table 3.2)
No- or low-fat salad dressing
(0 to 3 grams of fat per 2 dessertspoons)

2

Choice of salad, fruits, and vegetables
(unlimited quantity of the no-fat kind)
Choice of tuna, low-fat cottage cheese, sliced chicken
(1 to 3 grams of fat)
No- or low-fat salad dressing
(0 to 3 grams of fat per 2 dessertspoons)

3

Soup
(unlimited quantity of the no-fat kind)
Choice of sandwich
(1 gram of fat per slice of bread;
1 to 3 grams of fat per ounce/28 g of chicken or lean beef – see page 000;
plus unlimited greens, tomato, etc.;
ketchup and mustard have no fat;
4 grams of fat per scant teaspoon of mayonnaise)
Beverage

4

Unlimited fruit mixed in blender with
low- or very low-fat yoghurt
(no fat for fruit;
0 to 4 grams of fat for yoghurt)
Beverage

Compare the fat counts of these luncheon suggestions with the 53 grams of fat that are found in the fast-food restaurant versions of a *small* cheeseburger (31) and a *small* helping of chips (12).

What about soft drinks, with sugar or slimline? They don't contain fat, so are they permissible?

As a general rule, I don't approve of either. The sweetness of both keeps your sweet tooth alive and, in many people, leads to an over consumption of sweet FATTY foods. The intense sweetness also deadens your ability to appreciate natural sweetness in fruits and vegetables (there are 10 teaspoons of sugar in one 12 fl oz/330 ml cola drink). The diet varieties stimulate your system to expect honest-to-goodness calories, only nothing is there! This may stimulate appetite and lead to greater hunger than normal. (One important study showed that people who use diet drinks tend to end up gaining more weight over time than those who don't. It really pains me to see the consumption of diet drinks increasing so rapidly.) Both diet and sugary soft drinks may lead to a large insulin reaction that can block fat from leaving your fat cells temporarily, making it harder to lose fat weight.*

Now that I have said all this, I don't think an *occasional* soft drink or diet drink will harm you. However, if you are a slave to them, they may be playing a key role in your overeating of sweetened *fatty* foods. You will do much better if you switch to fruit juice, soda water or plain fresh water.

DINNER

I think you can see that breakfast and lunch combined can easily be designed to contain from 10 to 20 grams of fat. If you are a woman, this leaves half or more of your fat count of 20 to 40 grams available for the evening meal (men should add a little more fat to each meal because they are aiming for a total of 30 to 60 grams).

It is easy to design main courses of meat, fish, or poultry. Just see what you can do with lean cuts (fat grams for cooked portions):

Lean beef is about 2.5 grams of fat per ounce/28 g.
Breast of chicken (skinned) is about 1 gram of fat per ounce.
Dark meat of chicken (skinned) is 2.5 grams of fat per ounce.
Tenderloin of pork (the only lean on the pig) is 1 gram of fat per ounce.
Ham, lean and trimmed, is 3 grams of fat per ounce.

---

* Insulin helps move glucose out of the bloodstream into your body cells. Even though diet drinks contain no sugar they are capable of stimulating an insulin response in some people simply because of their sweet taste, just like regular soft drinks. A high circulating level of insulin signals your system that plenty of energy is present and tends to inhibit the mobilisation of fat from your fat cells. This is one reason people with hyperinsulinemia (high insulin levels) tend to have difficultly losing weight.

Fish (most varieties) is about *1 gram of fat per 4 ounces/110 g*.

Fatty varieties of fish (trout, salmon) are about 1 gram of fat per ounce.

High-fat cuts of meat can have two to three times the fat content of the lean cuts, and anything fried may have seven or eight times the fat content. Thus, if you build main courses around low-fat cuts you can eat a great deal of meat if you wish and still have a dinner containing under 20 grams of fat. That's impossible to do with fatty cuts. Add all the vegetables, potatoes, rice, other grains or pasta you want, plus fruit for dessert. Fat in the form of butter or margarine is 12 grams per desertspoon, so, when preparing vegetables, allow 1 dessertspoon of added fat for every serving for four – that's 3 grams per serving if none stuck to the pot. But I'll show you ways to cook many vegetables without any extra fat.

At cooked weights, 6 ounce/175 g portions of chicken and the leanest pork will amount to only 6 grams of fat, and fish is almost always much, much less. Six ounces of lean meat will contain about 12 grams of fat. If you add little or no fat to your vegetables you still have room for a slice of whole-grain bread or toast with honey or jam. A choice of fish, poultry, or a meatless dinner instead of beef will generally leave room for an ounce of Cheddar or some similar cheese (about 9 grams of fat) with fruit.

Here are a few suggestions for your main meal. Notice in my first suggestion how easy it is to think 'fat grams' and design a simple, basic Western-style meal containing only 20 grams of fat or less. Notice in the other selections how quickly and easily you can prepare different popular international dishes with minimum fat. These five dishes or styles of food preparation are basic for most people. You will find many different recipes for meat, fish, and fowl in the recipe chapter of this book (Chapter Six); and, while the main courses listed below suggest specific dishes and refer you to specific pages for the recipes, you will find several acceptable variations in the neighbouring pages of the recipe chapter.

1

Main course is choice of any of the
lean meats, fish or poultry, up to a
6 oz/175 g serving
(2 to 12 grams of fat)
Unlimited vegetables, potatoes, rice,
other grains, or legumes
(if fat added, 4 grams per scant teaspoon; no- or low-fat
salad dressings, 0 to 3 grams per 2 dessertspoons)

2
Main course is pasta
Choice of sauces (pages 137–40)
(4 to 12 grams of fat)
Large salad
(dressings, pages 149–50, fat grams 0 to 3)

3
Indian Spiced Beans, with rice,
topped with choice of chopped fresh vegetables, salsa and cheese
(1 gram of fat, page 133, plus 4 grams of fat
for each dessertspoon of grated cheese)

4
Pot Roast
(page 118; 12 grams of fat)
green salad or cooked green vegetables
compote of mixed dried fruit

5
Chilli-Bean Meat Loaf
(page 117; 9 grams of fat)
Large salad
(0 to 3 grams of fat for no- or low-fat dressings)

HOW TO USE THE T-FACTOR MENUS

The T-Factor Diet menus below are meant to introduce you to the wide variety of foods and styles of food preparation that will make your diet interesting and satisfying. Remember, however, that you can substitute any of the basic breakfasts and lunches listed above for the selections in these menus. You can substitute one vegetable for another, one fruit for another, one meat for another, etc. You don't need to follow the specific recipes that I recommend each day; instead, you may prepare any similar food in the manner I suggest in my other recipes in Chapter Six. You can alternate days or eat breakfast for dinner and dinner for breakfast if your day is normally topsy-turvy. Snacks can be eaten at any time of the day.

This flexibility may seem confusing to you at first. It is possible because – *assuming that you will eat a wide variety of foods from the different food groups* – the only nutrient that concerns us is FAT! When you control fat intake, keeping it within the 20- to 40-gram range if you are a woman and the 30- to 60-gram range if you're a man, you achieve an unbelieveable freedom in your choice of other foods. But if such flexibility confuses you at first, start by following the daily menus as closely as possible until you get a feeling for what this freedom implies.

USE THE FAT AND FIBRE COUNTER IN APPENDIX C WHEN YOU MAKE SUBSTITUTIONS.

KEEP TRACK OF FAT GRAMS EACH DAY IN THE MANNER I SUGGEST AT THE BEGINNING OF APPENDIX C.

ADD FAT-FREE FOODS AT MAIN MEALS OR FOR SNACKS UNTIL YOUR APPETITE IS SATISFIED. DON'T GO HUNGRY!

DAILY T-FACTOR MENUS

Many of these daily menus come out at the low end of the spectrum of 20 to 40 fat grams per day for women, leaving plenty of room for extra low-fat snacks or an occasional cake or pudding. Men may increase the portion sizes of the foods that contain fats by up to half to meet their goal of 30 to 60 grams of fat per day. For ease in counting, the fat-gram count in parentheses next to the foods listed (abbreviated for the menus as 'g') has been rounded up or down to the nearest whole gram in some instances.

Rice, pastas, and all vegetables are prepared without any added fat unless specified. Even if the package cooking directions call for fat in rice for example, just omit it; you won't miss it. When cereal is listed, I recommend a cereal mix. Try combining ½ oz/14 g of a high-fibre, high-bran-type cereal with ½ ounce of a more highly fortified cereal, such as Special K.

WEEK 1

[DAY I]

Breakfast   Banana or fresh fruit of choice; dry cereal (1 g per oz/28 g); 8 fl oz/225 ml of skimmed or low-fat milk (0–2 g); coffee or tea
Total fat: 1–3 g

Lunch   4 oz/110 g of low-fat cottage cheese (3 g); assorted raw vegetables; Ryvita (5 = 1 g); fresh fruit; no-cal beverage
Total fat: 4 g

Dinner   1 serving Baked Chicken with Tarragon and Fennel (page 127; 4 g) or 3½ oz/100 g roast chicken; brown or wild rice (1 g per serving); green beans; whole-grain bread (1 g per slice); tossed salad; no- or low-cal salad dressing (2 dessert-spoons = 0–3 g); fruit of choice; no-cal beverage
Total fat: 6–9 g

Snack	8 fl oz/225 ml plain, very low fat yoghurt; fresh strawberries; rice cakes (3 = 1 g)

Total fat: 1 g

Total fat for Day 1: 12–17 g

[DAY 2]

Breakfast	Grapefruit or fruit of choice; 1 egg, poached (5 g); whole-grain bread (1 g per slice); ½ teaspoon butter or margarine *or* 8 fl oz/225 ml skimmed milk (0–2 g); coffee or tea

Total fat: 6–8 g

Lunch	2 oz/56 g of sliced cooked chicken for sandwich (2 g); 2 slices of whole-grain bread (2 g); lettuce and sliced tomatoes; mustard; pear; no-cal beverage

Total fat: 4 g

Dinner	1 serving of Sea Bass with Red Peppers (page 113; 3 g); broccoli; tossed salad; no- or low-cal salad dressing (2 dessertspoons = 0–3 g); whole-grain bread (1 g per slice); fruit of choice; 1 serving of Cocoa Pudding Cake (page 156; 4 g); no-cal beverage

Total fat: 8–11 g

Snack	Dry cereal (1 g per oz/28 g); 1 cup of skimmed or low-fat milk (0–2 g); sliced fruit

Total fat: 1–3 g

Total fat for Day 2: 19–26 g

[DAY 3]

Breakfast	Honeydew melon or seasonal fruit; wholemeal bap (1 whole = 2 g); marmalade; 8 fl oz/225 ml low or very low fat plain yoghurt (0–2 g); coffee or tea

Total fat: 2–4 g

Lunch	2 oz/56 g of water-packed tuna (1 g); 1 scant teaspoon of mayonnaise (4 g); 1 roll (1 g); alfalfa sprouts and assorted raw vegetables; orange; no-cal beverage

Total fat: 6 g

Dinner	3 oz/80 g of Baked Flank Steak (page 116, 12 g); baked potato; green vegetable; tossed salad; no- or low-cal salad dressing (2 dessertspoons = 0–3 g); whole-grain bread (1 g per slice); fruit of choice, no-cal beverage

Total fat: 13–16 g

Snack	Fresh or dried fruit

Total fat: 0 g

Total fat for Day 3: 21–26 g

[DAY 4]

Breakfast   Dry cereal (1 g per oz/28 g); raisins; 8 fl oz/225 ml
skimmed or low fat milk (0–2 g); coffee or tea
    Total fat: 1–3 g

Lunch   Vegetable soup (2 g per 8 fl oz/225 ml); 1 tablespoon croutons (2 g); chef's salad of assorted raw
vegetables, 1 oz/28 g of turkey (1 g), ½ oz/14 g of
hard cheese (4–5 g); no- or low-cal salad dressing
(2 dessertspoons = 0–3 g); apple; no-cal beverage
    Total fat: 9–13 g

Dinner   1 helping of spaghetti (2 g) with 8 fl oz/225 ml
Meat Sauce (page 139; 12 g); steamed courgettes;
whole-grain bread (1 g per slice); fresh fruit;
no-cal beverage
    Total fat: 15 g

Snack   8 fl oz/225 ml very low fat yoghurt; banana; water
3 rice cakes (1 g)
    Total fat: 1 g
    Total fat for Day 4: 26–32 g

[DAY 5]

Breakfast   Assorted fresh fruit; porridge or other hot cereal
(1 g per 4 fl oz/110 ml); 8 fl oz/225 ml skimmed or
low-fat milk (0–2 g); whole-grain toast (1 g per
slice); marmalade; coffee or tea
    Total fat: 2–4 g

Lunch   Toasted pitta pocket: 6-inch/15 cm whole-grain
pitta (1 g), 1 oz/28 g of shredded hard cheese
(8–10 g), sliced tomato, assorted raw vegetables;
orange or grapefruit; no-cal beverage
    Total fat: 9–11 g

Dinner   1 serving of Simple Fish in Foil (page 114; 1.5 g)
or 4 oz/110 g of sole or plaice, sliced onions, carrots,
potatoes and green beans (1.5 g); whole-grain
bread (1 g per slice); 1 serving of Lemon Meringue Pie (page 157; 6 g) or Chocolate Meringue Pie
(page 155, 6 g); no-cal beverage
    Total fat: 8½ g

Snack   Dry cereal (1 g/28 g per oz); 8 fl oz/225 ml skimmed or low-fat milk (0–2 g); sliced fresh fruit
    Total fat: 1–3 g
    Total fat for Day 5: 20½–26½ g

[DAY 6]

Breakfast   Seasonal fruit; 1 roll (1 g); honey; ½ teaspoon
butter or margarine *or* 8 fl oz/225 ml skimmed
milk (0–2 g); coffee or tea
Total fat: 1–3 g

Lunch   2 oz/56 g of sliced turkey for sandwich (2 g);
2 slices of whole-grain bread (2 g); lettuce and
tomato slices; mustard; apple; no-cal beverage
Total fat: 4 g

Dinner   Basic Better Beans (page 131; 5 g per 4 oz/110 g
serving); brown rice (1 g per serving); spinach or
other greens; Massachusetts Corn Muffin (page
95; 3 g each); tossed salad; no- or low-cal salad
dressing (2 dessertspoons = 0–3 g); fresh fruit;
no-cal beverage
Total fat: 9–12 g

Snack   Fresh fruit; 3 rice cakes (1 g)
Total fat: 1 g
Total fat for Day 6: 15–20 g

[DAY 7]

Breakfast   Grapefruit or fruit of choice; dry cereal (1 g per
oz/28 g); 8 fl oz/225 ml skimmed or low-fat milk
(0–2 g); coffee or tea
Total fat: 1–3 g

Lunch   Minestrone (page 108, 1 g per serving); Massachusetts Corn Muffin (page 95; 3 g); peach or
pear; no-cal beverage
Total fat: 4 g

Dinner   3 oz/80 g of lean, well-trimmed pork loin (9 g);
Apple-Sweet Potatoes (page 141; 1 g per serving);
tossed salad; no- or low-cal salad dressing (2 dessertspoons = 0–3 g); whole-grain bread (1 g per
slice); fruit of choice; no-cal beverage
Total fat: 11–14 g

Snack   8 fl oz/225 ml very low fat plain yoghurt; sliced
banana; 5 Ryvita (1 g)
Total fat: 1 g
Total fat for Day 7: 17–22 g

WEEK 2

Breakfast Seasonal fruit; plain, very low fat yoghurt; high-fibre cereal (1 g per ounce; stir in with yoghurt and fruit); whole-grain bread (1 g per slice); coffee or tea
 Total fat: 2 g

Lunch 2 oz/56 g of sliced turkey (2 g); whole-grain bread (1 g per slice); lettuce and tomato slices; mustard and cress; orange; no-cal beverage
 Total fat: 3 g

Dinner 4½ oz/125 g of Royal Indian Salmon (page 111; 8 g); green beans; brown or wild rice (1 g per 4 oz/110 g); tossed salad; no- or low-cal salad dressing (2 dessertspoons = 0–3 g); whole-grain bread (1 g per slice); fruit of choice; no-cal beverage
 Total fat: 10–13 g

Snack 8 fl oz/225 ml skimmed or low-fat milk (0–2 g); crispbread (2–4 = 1 g); apple
 Total fat: 1–3 g
 Total fat for Day 8: 16–21 g

Breakfast Sliced banana; dry cereal (1 g per oz/28 g); 8 fl oz/ 225 ml skimmed or low-fat milk (0–2 g); coffee or tea
 Total fat: 1–3 g

Lunch 2 oz/56 g of water-packed tuna (1 g); 1 scant tea-spoon of mayonnaise (4 g); whole-grain pitta pocket (½ = 1 g); assorted raw vegetables; grape-fruit or orange; no-cal beverage
 Total fat: 6 g

Dinner 1 serving of Salmon Croquettes Béarnaise (5½ g); boiled potatoes; frozen peas or other green vegetable; tossed salad; no- or low-cal salad dressing (2 desertspoons = 0–3 g); 1 serv-ing of Cocoa Pudding Cake (page 156; 4 g); no-cal beverage
 Total fat: 9½–12½ g

Snack Fresh or dried fruit
 Total fat: 0 g
 Total fat for Day 9: 16½–21½ g

[DAY 10]

Breakfast Fresh fruit of choice; bap (1 whole = 2 g); honey; ½ teaspoon butter or margarine *or* 8 fl oz/225 ml skimmed milk (0–2 g); coffee or tea
  Total fat: 2–4 g

Lunch Chicken noodle soup: 1 oz/28 g of diced, cooked chicken, small serving (about 3 oz/80 g) noodles, diced vegetables, chicken bouillon (2 g); Applesauce-Bran Muffin (page 94; 3 g); apple; no-cal beverage
  Total fat: 5 g

Dinner 1 serving of Light and Easy Lemon Chicken (page 129; 4 g) or 3½ oz/95 g of chicken breast; steamed courgettes, young turnip and green peppers; brown rice (4 oz/110 g cooked = 1 g); tossed salad; no- or low-cal salad dressing (2 dessertspoons = 0–3 g); whole-grain bread (1 g per slice); fruit of choice; 1 serving of Poppy-Seed Cake (page 158; 7 g); no-cal beverage
  Total fat: 16 g

Snack 8 fl oz/225 ml very low fat plain yoghurt; sliced peaches; dry cereal (1 g per ounce)
  Total fat: 1 g
  Total fat for Day 10: 21–26 g

[DAY 11]

Breakfast Fresh fruit of choice; dry cereal (1 g per oz/28 g); 8 fl oz/225 ml skimmed or low-fat milk (0–2 g); coffee or tea
  Total fat: 1–3 g

Lunch Spinach salad: fresh spinach, sliced fresh mushrooms, ½ hard-boiled egg (3 g), ½ oz/14 g low-fat white cheese (4 g), chopped onions, no- or low-cal salad dressing (2 dessertspoons = 0–3 g); Applesauce-Bran Muffin (page 94; 3 g); orange; no-cal beverage
  Total fat: 10–13 g

Dinner 4½ oz/125 g of Baked Turkey Loaf (page 127; 12 g); fresh steamed broccoli; baked marrow; tossed salad; no- or low-cal salad dressing (2 dessertspoons = 0–3 g); whole-grain bread (1 g per slice); apple; no-cal beverage
  Total fat: 13–16 g

Snack Fresh fruit
  Total fat: 0 g
  Total fat for Day 11: 24–32 g

[DAY 12]

Breakfast   Honeydew melon or other seasonal fruit; 1 egg cooked without fat (5 g); whole-grain toast (1 g per slice); ½ teapoon butter or margarine *or* 8 fl oz/225 ml skimmed milk (0–2 g); coffee or tea
Total fat: 6–8 g

Lunch   3 oz/80 g of leftover Baked Turkey Loaf for sandwich (8 g); 1 whole-grain roll (2 g); lettuce and tomato slices; grapes; no-cal beverage
Total fat: 10 g

Dinner   1 serving of Spinach Lasagna (page 135, 8 g) or Aubergine Parmesan (page 133; 8 g – add 4 oz/110 g cooked pasta (2 g) with Aubergine Parmesan); whole-grain roll (2 g); tossed salad, no- or low-cal salad dressing (2 dessertspoons = 0–3 g); fresh fruit; no-cal beverage
Total fat: 10–14 g

Snack   Dry cereal (1 g per ounce/28 g); 8 fl oz/225 ml skimmed or low-fat milk (0–2 g); banana
Total fat: 1–3 g
Total fat for Day 12: 27–35 g

[DAY 13]

Breakfast   Porridge or other hot cereal (1 g per serving); sultanas; dash of cinnamon; 8 fl oz/225 ml skimmed or low-fat milk (0–2 g); coffee or tea
Total fat: 1–3 g

Lunch   2 oz/56 g tinned salmon (4 g); 1 scant teaspoon mayonnaise (4 g); 1 whole-grain roll (1 g); alfalfa sprouts and assorted raw vegetables; pear; no-cal beverage
Total fat: 9 g

Dinner   3 oz/80 g of Round-Roast Oriental (page 119; 9 g); baked potato; Brussels Sprouts with Caraway Seeds (page 143; 1 serving = 1 g) or other green vegetable; whole-grain bread (1 g per slice); tossed salad; no- or low-cal salad dressing (2 dessertspoons = 0–3 g); fresh fruit; no-cal beverage
Total fat: 11–14 g

Snack   8 fl oz/225 ml very low fat plain yoghurt; fresh strawberries or other fruit; 3 rice cakes (1 g)
Total fat: 1 g
Total fat for Day 13: 22–27 g

Breakfast   Grapefruit; 1 roll (2 g); honey; ½ teaspoon butter
             or margarine *or* 8 fl oz/225 ml skimmed milk
             (0–2 g); coffee or tea
                  Total fat: 1–3 g

Lunch   4 oz/110 g low-fat cottage cheese (3 g); assorted
             fresh fruit; Ryvita or other whole-grain crispbread
             (5 = 1 g); assorted raw vegetables; no-cal
             beverage
                  Total fat: 4 g

Dinner   Broccoli Soup (page 107; 8 fl oz/225 ml = 3 g); 1
             serving of Grilled Tuna Mediterranean (page 110;
             9 g); steamed carrots; brown or wild rice (1 g);
             whole-grain bread (1 g per slice); fresh fruit;
             no-cal beverage
                  Total fat: 14 g

Snack   Dry cereal (1 g per oz/28 g; 8 fl oz/225 ml skim-
             med or low-fat milk (0–2 g); fresh fruit
                  Total fat: 1–3 g
                  Total fat for Day 14: 20–24 g

WEEK 3

[DAY 15]

Breakfast   Banana; dry cereal (1 g per oz/28 g); 8 fl oz/
             225 ml skimmed or low-fat milk (0–2 g); coffee
             or tea
                  Total fat: 1–3 g

Lunch   Tuna-stuffed tomato: 2–3 oz/56–80 g of water-
             packed tuna (1 g), 1 scant teaspoon mayonnaise
             (4 g), chopped celery, whole tomato; Ryvita or
             other whole-grain crispbread (5 = 1 g); orange;
             no-cal beverage
                  Total fat: 6 g

Dinner   1 serving of Quick Turkey Chop Suey (page 130;
             8 g); brown or wild rice (1 g per serving); whole-
             wheat roll (1 roll = 2 g); tossed salad; no- or
             low-cal salad dressing (2 dessertspoons = 0–3 g);
             1 serving of Elegant Pears (page 156; 2 g); no-cal
             beverage
                  Total fat: 13–16 g

Snack   8 fl oz/225 ml very low fat yoghurt; fresh fruit of
             choice; 3 rice cakes (1 g)
                  Total fat: 1 g
                  Total fat for Day 15: 21–26 g

[DAY 16]

Breakfast Grapefruit; bap (1 whole = 2 g); marmalade; ½
teaspoon butter or margarine *or* 8 fl oz/225 ml
skimmed milk (0–2 g); coffee or tea
Total fat: 2–4 g

Lunch 2 oz/56 g cooked chicken (2 g); whole-grain
bread (1 g per slice); lettuce and sliced tomatoes;
mustard; pretzels (1 oz/28 g = 1 g); apple; no-cal
beverage
Total fat: 4 g

Dinner 3 oz/80 g Swedish Meatballs (page 121; 14 g);
brown, wild, or saffron rice (1 serving = 1 g);
green beans; tossed salad; no- or low-cal salad
dressing (2 dessertspoons = 0–3 g); whole-grain
bread (1 g per slice); fresh fruit; no-cal beverage
Total fat: 16–19 g

Snack Fresh or dried fruit
Total fat 0 g
Total fat for Day 16: 22–27 g

[DAY 17]

Breakfast Porridge or other hot cereal (1 g per serving);
raisins; whole-grain bread (1 g per slice); honey;
½ teaspoon butter or margarine *or* 8 fl oz/225 ml
skimmed milk (0–2 g); coffee or tea
Total fat: 2–4 g

Lunch Home-made vegetable-type soup (8 fl oz/225 ml
= 2 g); chef's salad: assorted raw vegetables,
1 oz/28 g of turkey, ½ oz/14 g of hard cheese
(5 g); no- or low-cal salad dressing (2 dessertspoons = 0–3 g); Ryvita (5 = 1 g); pear;
no-cal beverage
Total fat: 8–11 g

Dinner 1 serving of Vegetable Stroganoff (page 135; 2 g)
with average helping of cooked grain or pasta (2 g);
whole-grain roll (1 2-inch roll = 2 g); tossed salad;
no- or low-cal salad dressing (2 dessertspoons =
0–3 g); fresh fruit with Sweet Yoghurt Dressing
(page 150; 1½ g); no-cal beverage
Total fat: 7½–10½ g

Snack Dry cereal (1 g per oz/28 g); sliced fresh fruit; 8 fl
oz/225 ml skimmed or low-fat milk (0–2 g)
Total fat: 1–3 g
Total fat for Day 17: 16½–28½ g

Breakfast Fresh fruit of choice; dry cereal (1 g per oz/28 g); 8 fl oz/225 ml skimmed or low-fat milk (0–2 g); coffee or tea
Total fat: 1–3 g

Lunch 4 oz/110 g seasoned low-fat cottage cheese (3 g); 1 roll (1 g); alfalfa sprouts and raw vegetables; assorted fresh fruit; no-cal beverage
Total fat: 4 g

Dinner 1 serving of Pork Chops Parmesan (page 125; 12 g); cooked cauliflower; unsweetened apple sauce; spinach noodles (1 serving = 1 g); tossed salad; no- or low-cal salad dressing (2 tablespoons = 0–3 g); whole-grain bread (1 g per slice); fresh fruit; no-cal beverage
Total fat: 14–17 g

Snack 8 fl oz/225 ml very low fat plain yoghurt; fresh fruit of choice; 3 rice cakes (1 g)
Total fat: 1 g
Total fat for Day 18: 20–25 g

[DAY 19]

Breakfast Fresh fruit of choice; 1 roll (1 g); marmalade; 8 fl oz/225 ml skimmed or low-fat milk (0–2 g); coffee or tea
Total fat: 1–3 g

Lunch 2 oz/56 g sliced turkey for sandwich (2 g); 2 slices whole-grain bread (2 g); lettuce and tomato slices; mustard and cress; pretzels (1 oz/28 g = 1 g); strawberries or seasonal fruit; no-cal beverage
Total fat: 5 g

Dinner Basic Better Beans (page 131; 1 serving = 5 g); rice; bulghur wheat or whole-grain pasta (1 serving = 1–2 g); chopped onions and peppers; lettuce and assorted raw vegetables; low- or no-cal dressing (2 dessertspoons = 0-3 g); ½ oz/14 g or 2 dessertspoons grated cheese (5 g); apple; no-cal beverage
Total fat: 11–15 g

Snack Fresh or dried fruit
Total fat: 0 g
Total fat for Day 19: 17–23 g

Breakfast Grapefruit; 1 egg, cooked without fat (5 g); whole-grain toast (1 g per slice); ½ teaspoon butter or margarine *or* 8 fl oz/225 ml skimmed milk (0–2 g); coffee or tea
    Total fat: 6–8 g

Lunch Home-made vegetable soup (8 fl oz/225 ml = 0-2 g); Ginger-snap Muffin (page 95; 3 g); assorted raw vegetables; grapes; no-cal beverage
    Total fat: 3–5 g

Dinner 3½ oz/95 g Barbecued Chicken (page 128; 5 g); 1 serving of Scalloped Potatoes (page 144; 4 g); steamed seasoned courgettes; tossed salad; no- or low-cal salad dressing (2 dessertspoons = 0–3 g); whole-grain bread (1 g per slice); fresh fruit; no-cal beverage
    Total fat: 10–13 g

Snack Dry cereal (1 g per oz/28 g); banana; 8 fl oz/ 225 ml skimmed or low-fat milk (0–2 g)
    Total fat: 1–3 g
    Total fat for Day 20: 20–29 g

Breakfast Sliced fresh fruit; dry cereal (1 g per oz/28 g); 8 fl oz/225 ml skimmed or low-fat milk (0–2 g); coffee or tea
    Total fat: 1–3 g

Lunch Toasted pitta pocket: whole-grain pitta (1 g), 1 oz/28 g shredded hard cheese (8–10 g), sliced tomato, assorted raw vegetables; orange; no-cal beverage
    Total fat: 9–11 g

Dinner 1 serving of Shrimps Florentine (page 113; 7 g) or 3–4 oz/80–110 g grilled fish and green vegetable; brown or wild rice (1 serving = 1 g); whole-grain bread (1 g per slice); apple; no-cal beverage
    Total fat: 9 g

Snack 8 fl oz/225 ml very low fat plain yoghurt; sliced peaches; 3 rice cakes (1 g)
    Total fat: 1 g
    Total fat for Day 21: 20–24 g

CHAPTER FOUR

WHAT TO EXPECT WHEN YOU USE THE T-FACTOR DIET

As I reported in Chapter Two, the overweight women who used the basic fat-gram formula of the T-Factor Diet, without making any effort to count or cut calories, achieved an average weight loss of slightly over 7 pounds (3 kg) during the first three weeks of the diet and around a pound (450 g) a week thereafter. Two of the women lost a pound a day the first week, but obviously it would be nearly impossible to lose that much fat weight so quickly. These women had been retaining a great deal of water and they lost it when they began the diet.

However, all the women in the group started off with a bang because, as is generally the case, the speed of weight loss correlates with existing weight. Even without making an effort to cut calories, women who are as overweight as they were, and retaining water, can lose as much as a pound a day in the first few days of the T-Factor Diet. From then on, the weight loss will reflect the difference between your fat intake and the fat you burn in your fuel mixture.

In this chapter I want to report some of the experiences that people have had with the diet, especially those of a young married couple who were among the first to test the diet more than a year ago. Both husband and wife have each lost more than 3½ stone (23 kg) and kept them off. I will talk about this couple later in the chapter because they illustrate what a family can do when it works together.

WHAT ABOUT 'FINAL 5 TO 15'?

But what about those people who have only 5 to 15 pounds (2 to 7 kg) to lose? What can they expect? Those final 5 to 15 are often the hardest pounds to lose. They are a source of aggravation and distress for millions of people throughout their lives.

As I reported in Chapter Two, the T-Factor Diet proved to be 100 per cent successful with a group of young women who had been struggling with this small amount of excess fat and who went on the diet after hearing about it on a health promotion course. By losing an average of 5 pounds (2 kg), the group's average weight is now right in the middle of the band suggested on the charts.

In addition to these women, the entire professional staff of the Vanderbilt Weight Management Program has also adopted the T-Factor Diet. I want in particular to report the experiences that Ms Jamie Pope-Cordle, director of nutrition in the Vanderbilt Weight Management Program, and I have had with the diet. We both fit the 'final 5 to 15' category, and we kept records of our experience. We will talk about ourselves first, and then report the experiences of heavier participants in the Vanderbilt Program.

MY EXPERIENCE IMPLEMENTING THE T-FACTOR DIET

I couldn't possibly recommend a diet that I hadn't tried myself, especially when the diet is supposed to embody health-enhancing principles that I recommend you follow for the rest of your life.

So I did exactly what I suggest you do, with the intention of making a lifetime life-style change. Here is my personal report.

I surveyed my current eating habits to determine how much fat I was eating. I counted fat grams. At first, I often had to look them up.

To my surprise, I was eating, on average, about 100 grams of fat a day. Now, I am normally a very active person – jogging or playing tennis just about every day. Before adopting the T-Factor Diet I ate on average about 3,000 calories a day to maintain my weight at around 11½ stone (72 kg), which, at 5 feet 10½ inches, is smack in the middle of the range of suggested weight in the charts. (If you have read my previous books you will know that I lost over 5 stone (34 kg) twenty-five years ago and have never regained that weight.) One hundred grams of fat is about 30 per cent of my total intake and most experts would consider that percentage of calories in fat well within the healthy range. As an absolute amount, however, it is far more than necessary for good health.

When I decided to begin living by the principles of the T-Factor Diet, I wanted the answers to several questions:

1. If I cut back to 60 grams of fat per day and ate freely of

anything I wanted in the carbohydrate category, would I lose weight?

2. Considering that I was making no effort to cut calories, how fast would I lose?

3. If I adopted the T-Factor Diet permanently, where would my weight stabilize? I didn't think that I could afford to lose more than 5 or 10 pounds (2 to 4 kg). On the one occasion when I fell below a weight of 10 stone 10 pounds (68 kg) after spending two weeks on an experimental very-low-calorie diet, I didn't feel well and my friends and colleagues all remarked on my poor appearance.

4. Where was the fat coming from in my current diet, and if I cut back, would I be able to make healthy substitutions and end up with a better choice of foods?

5. How would I feel?

6. Would I enjoy it?

7. Would I be able to continue eating in my favourite restaurants?

THE CHANGES I MADE

When I surveyed my eating habits looking for the excess fat calories, two things stood out: cheese and mayonnaise.

Since I don't care for milk as a beverage and, except for butter and cream, other dairy products in general are good to excellent sources of calcium, I had chosen cheese as my primary calcium-containing food. But I was eating as much as 4 to 6 ounces (110 to 175 g) a day, using varieties like Cheddar or havarti when I made cheese toast or cheese sandwiches.

Before you read any further, do you know the fat-gram count in 4 to 6 ounces of Cheddar cheese? We're talking 36 to 54 grams of fat, or 324 to 486 calories from fat in the cheese component of my daily diet. I had not realized how that one food item, all by itself, made up the major part of my fat intake each day.

As to the mayonnaise, on the two or three days each week when I made sandwiches using mayonnaise – well, let's just say I've had a love affair with mayonnaise all my life! When I was a fat adolescent, I would sneak down to the kitchen at night and have mayonnaise sandwiches, with or without onions, on thick slices of pumpernickel bread. To this day, I really like mayonnaise, and I was spreading each sandwich with at least a tablespoonful and eating two at a sitting. I might finish up with a slice or two of bread and mayonnaise after eating the two sandwiches. That's another 24 to 36 grams of fat – or 216 to 324 calories.

In other words, about half the fat in my diet was coming from these two sources, cheese and mayonnaise!

When you survey your own eating habits I think you, too, will find that a major part of the fat in your diet derives from just two, or possibly three, sources. It's not hard to change once you've located the main culprits because so many healthy substitutions are possible.

This is what I did.

About six out of seven days a week I began to substitute either cereal and low-fat milk for the cheese toast or a generous helping of variously seasoned low-fat cottage cheese* with a roll or whole-grain toast. Thus, even with two bowls of cereal, with fruit such as a banana, a cup of berries or a sliced peach, and with 8 fluid ounces (225 ml) of low-fat milk, I was at 6 to 8 grams of fat, not 36 to 54. A whole carton of low-fat cottage cheese, which I most frequently began to eat with a variety of different spicy salsas in place of the hard cheeses, also comes to about 6 grams of fat. Whenever I did eat Cheddar or other hard cheeses that are high in fat I made sure it was never over 2 ounces (56 g) a day. In order to guarantee that I was getting enough calcium I increased my consumption of leafy greens and other vegetables such as broccoli, and made sure I ate sardines, tinned salmon or tinned mackerel once a week. These tinned fishes are good sources of calcium because they contain the bones in edible form.

Then I discovered something about mayonnaise. When I cut back to a scant teaspoonful I found that within a couple of days my sensitivity to its taste increased to the point where even a small amount became perfectly satisfying. So, my mayonnaise consumption was cut by two-thirds. I think I was able to cut my consumption of mayonnaise and still enjoy the limited amounts because I continued to use my favourite, full-flavoured brands rather than low-calorie substitutes.

You can see that saving over 40 grams of fat in cheese and mayonnaise wasn't all that difficult for me, and I'll bet that you will find similar 'savings' are possible in your own case. Here is a short summary of some other things that permitted me to cut my fat grams substantially and end up with an even healthier diet than before:

When I didn't have cereal or cottage cheese for breakfast, I had hearty whole-grain bread, rolls or home-made muffins (pages 94–98) and, on occasion, the very best marmalades and jams. I found it hard to believe I could be eating toast and marmalade and losing weight.

---

* Be sure to try my suggestions on page 99 for flavouring this old standby. Never before did I find cottage cheese to be a particularly inviting food, but these seasonings have made it one of my favourites.

Instead of sandwiches for lunch, spread with that blanket of mayonnaise, I began to eat much more soup (pages 105–9) and cottage cheese, if I hadn't had it for breakfast. When I did make sandwiches, I used one-third my previous amount of mayonnaise. At times I skipped the mayonnaise completely and began to use more different-flavoured mustards. When having lunch close to the university, I found three restaurants that served a variety of salads, soups, and sandwiches where I could choose lunches totalling 10 grams of fat or less. At our suggestion, one of the restaurants began serving at least one 'non-cream' home-made soup each day, to go with sliced turkey or lean-meat sandwiches, all made without mayonnaise, but with a variety of mustards. All we had to do was make the suggestion to the owner.

I increased my number of meatless meals for dinner (pages 131–6), and made many more interesting fish and poultry recipes (pages 110–115 and 127–30). But I still had beef about once a week, since I do enjoy a well-seasoned steak (page 121) or pot roast (page 118).

HOW FAST DID I LOSE?

SLOWLY!!

As I have said before, on the basic T-Factor Diet people who are significantly overweight will lose much more quickly than I did. If you are in the 'final 5 to 15' category, you too, like myself, may face the prospect of a slow (but certain) weight loss.

If I had been in a hurry to lose weight I would have used the Quick Melt. I already know from experimenting with other low-calorie diets that I can lose up to nine pounds (4 kg) in two weeks if I cut my calories down to the Quick Melt levels. After finishing the experimental diet, however, I would resume my old eating habits and my weight would return to its former level.

This time I wanted to experience the real test of nutrient substitution, and see where my weight would end up when I simply changed the proportion of fat in my diet. *This was not going to be a weight-loss diet. It was an experiment to determine whether I could make a lifetime change in my eating habits – the kind of change that's necessary for those who want to lose weight and keep it off permanently. Would this change lead to an automatic downward adjustment in my weight?*

I lost:

Week 1	½ lb/225 g
Week 2	½ lb/225 g
Week 3	½ lb/225 g
Week 4	1½ lb/675 g
Week 5	2¼ lb/1,010 g
Week 6	1 lb/450 g
Week 7	1 lb/450 g

By the eighth week I stabilized at this new level.

I learned several things about losing weight in this fashion rather than by 'going on a diet' and some of the following details may be of help to you as you lose your 'final 5 to 15' on the T-Factor Diet.

My weight would frequently fluctuate as much as 2 pounds (1 kg) a day. It was 2 pounds up after each of the two times we went out for dinner in a Chinese restaurant (we ask for our food to be prepared without monosodium glutamate, but there is plenty of sodium from table salt in commercially prepared Chinese food even without the MSG). My weight was up a pound when I had pickles – which is why I warn people, 'It's a pound a pickle.' It was up 2 pounds after an Italian dinner, with wine. Remember this about alcohol: It has a slight diuretic effect in the short term, but many people rebound and rehydrate beyond their baseline water balance. They end up retaining water and weighing more than they did before, twelve to twenty-four hours after drinking any alcohol.

All these temporary increases that I mention were superimposed on a slowly descending baseline, but if I had got on the scales every day expecting to see myself lighter I would have been terribly disappointed. I weighed myself only to see the impact on my water balance, knowing that I was losing fat weight even if it was not detected by the scales.

SO – UNLESS YOU HAVE A SCIENTIFIC INTEREST IN WATCHING YOUR WEIGHT FLUCTUATIONS, I SUGGEST YOU WEIGH YOURSELF NO MORE THAN ONCE A WEEK. IF THAT!

Perhaps the very best way to implement the T-Factor Diet is to forget about the scales completely. Throw them away so that you will never be their slave again. Trust your body and Mother Nature. If you follow a healthy diet and activity programme, the weight will take care of itself.

But why did I have the sudden loss in the fourth and fifth weeks? First, I had started rather slowly. Second, in some people, there is a tendency for fat cells to take in a bit of water to replace the fat they lose at the beginning of any weight-loss programme. This water is sometimes held for several weeks. Then, suddenly, out it goes. Third, in those two weeks of quicker losses, I may have weighed myself at a low point in my water balance. I hit a plateau in Week 7, and from then on my weight has bounced around this new low point.

HOW DID I FEEL?

Great! I certainly wouldn't be writing about it if I didn't find myself feeling more energetic than before – and I was building on a rather high baseline since I had felt fine on my previous diet. People remarked spontaneously how good I looked and how energetic I seemed. This turns out to be a common experience among those who switch to the T-Factor Diet.

DID I EAT AS MUCH AS BEFORE?

I could not give this a good test at first because I sustained a knee injury playing tennis and was not able to jog or play tennis for fourteen weeks. My calorie intake dropped to about 2,400 a day from 3,000. BUT THAT LED TO AN INTERESTING, DIFFERENT KIND OF TEST, WHICH PROVED THAT WEIGHT LOSS WAS POSSIBLE, IN FACT QUITE EASY, WITHOUT MY USUAL LEVEL OF ACTIVITY.

Because weight loss occurred automatically with the cutback in fat intake, in spite of my inability to continue my customary physical activities, I feel that the T-Factor Diet offers hope to people who have physical limitations on the amount of exercise they can pursue. We have not given this a formal test because we feel that exercise is very important to good health, but we have worked with a few individuals who are not able to exercise consistently for one reason or another, with good results, as you will see from my discussion below.

As my injury healed, I gradually resumed jogging, going from short stints to one to three miles, two to three times a week, back up to full steam, mixing five or six miles of jogging on alternate days with tennis. Just as the experts predict, my caloric intake increased approximately 100 calories per mile of activity. (In tennis, according to actual measurements made on many occasions. I move almost exactly five miles in every 1½ hours of singles play.) I now eat a few more grams of fat each day, but the major part of that extra intake is in carbohydrate foods.

THE T-FACTOR DIET IS LIVABLE

I found that within the few weeks my low-fat for high-fat substitutions became second nature. Today, I no longer think about it. I've become used to small amounts of fat and even the thought of increasing makes me feel a little nauseated. I would find it hard to resume my old way of eating. You, too, will discover how much easier it is to digest low-fat meals and how much better you will feel as you follow the T-Factor Diet.

EATING OUT

I have already mentioned how I deal with lunches when I eat out close to the university. Most of the restaurants where we like to eat dinner have several low-fat dishes on their menus. Look around your own city for restaurants that offer good low-fat cooking. There is so much interest developing in eating a more healthy diet that more and more restaurants are responding and making it possible to eat out without pigging it.

But in those few cases where suitable things do not appear on the menu, ASK! One of my favourite restaurants *never* prepares anything on its menu without 2 ounces (56 g) of butter or a rich cream sauce. The owner to this day feels than when people go out to eat they want to kill themselves with 'goodness'. Yet the excellent chef at this restaurant will make anything I ask for without the fat or cream, and if I want a taste of the sauce he will serve it separately. Any decent restaurant should be happy to do the same for you. It's important to overcome your embarrassment about asking for special food preparation; in a recent American survey, 75 per cent of restaurants said they would modify their manner of food preparation on request.

If you have any doubt about the restaurant's willingness to prepare food the way you want it, telephone and ask them in advance. Just about all fish, poultry, veal, and beef can be prepared without added fat. At the most, a touch of oil is all it takes to prevent sticking and to keep the food tender. When it comes to pasta, plain tomato sauce will generally be lowest in fat. *Except for fast-food establishments, I personally have never found a restaurant that would not make one or more dishes in the low-fat manner that I prefer if I could not find something on the menu.*

THE T-FACTOR EXPERIENCE:
A NUTRITIONIST'S VIEWPOINT

Ms Jamie Pope-Cordle is the director of nutrition for the Vanderbilt Weight Management Program. She, like me, fits into that 'final 5 to 15' category. She gave me this summary at a Thanksgiving Day dinner in 1988 of her experience using the T-Factor approach.

I can remember my freshman year in college and my first nutrition course: 'Whether you eat it as chocolate cake or celery, a calorie is a calorie – carbohydrate, fat and protein created equal.' There was no reason to debate the issue. In the mid-seventies scientific evidence did not exist that pinpointed fat as the crucial factor in weight management. The research and clinical findings concerning differences in the metabolism, storage and mobilization of fat and carbohydrate have only been brought to the scientific community's attention in the last few years. The vast majority of nutrition texts still do not reflect these findings.

I have been a chronic calorie counter ever since that 1975 freshman nutrition course. Battling my own weight against a family history of obesity and a mild obsession with food, I became a walking calculator – I rarely went to sleep without a daily inventory of calories consumed and expended. I was even known to count the calories of people in front of me at checkout tills, silently comparing their caloric purchases with mine. Sounds crazy, but I bet this hits home with a few others as well!

So, needless to say, switching from counting calories to counting fat grams was quite a switch. I had to add another automatic function to my mental calculator. I started counting fat grams a little over three months ago, although I have been aware of the 'proportion' of calories from fat for several years. I had always strived to keep my own intake of fat, along with that of participants in my weight-management programmes at Vanderbilt, to less than 30 per cent of total calories. However, the importance of a specific number of fat grams became evident to me as I did research for a grant proposal concerning low-fat reducing diets. In addition, we began to notice that participants in our own studies who made the greatest reduction in their fat intake lost the most weight. Of course, calorie reduction facilitated the loss, but fat intake seemed to be the most significant factor. Those who ate the same 'type' of diet as they had previously, that is, choosing the same high-fat foods but in smaller quantities to achieve caloric reduction, did not do as well as those who switched their eating style to lower-fat higher-fibre fare.

When I first started counting fat grams I found I still couldn't resist a nightly calorie inventory. At the beginning, on some days, despite eating three meals and two snacks, I found I was eating only 1,300 calories. I lost 5 pounds (2 kg) in two and a half weeks even though I intentionally tried to increase my intake to at least 1,800 calories per day. The weight loss just 'happened' after I began stocking my kitchen with a brand-new variety of low-fat foods. I was rather surprised, though, that I lost this much weight because I was even testing recipes for the book during this period, which meant lots of taste testing.

In the past I used to average around 1,800 calories a day and I maintained my weight with running and walking fifteen to twenty miles a week. Now my weight has stabilized at 4 pounds lower than when I started and I have increased my intake to around 2,000 calories a day. But I cringe to reveal, as of late, I have not been exercising at that same level. Normally, this would have shown up as a few extra pounds on my thighs and stomach. I am confident that I would have seen my weight stabilize at an even lower point if I had been consistent in my activity *and* that I would be eating around 2,200 calories and weighing less. It is obvious to me that not only can I eat more food in terms of volume and weight, but in calories, too, as long as they are carbohydrate calories and not fat calories.

And, just for your information, I don't know how many calories I ate today – I don't add them up any more. I had 34 grams of fat – but I am not really counting fat grams any more either. You just learn how to eat differently.

A FINAL WORD ON THE 'FINAL 5 TO 15'

The T-Factor Diet is *the* certain way to eliminate the final 5 to 15 pounds you may have been struggling with for years. Just as in my own case, and as with the young women whose results I reported in Chapter Two, fat loss may proceed at about 1 to 1½ pounds (450 to 675 g) a week rather than at the faster rate that significantly overweight people achieve. But, just as our follow-up with these women showed, WE ARE TALKING ABOUT 100 PER CENT SUCCESS WITH *YOUR* FINAL 5 TO 15 POUNDS WHEN YOU STICK WITH THE T-FACTOR FAT-GRAM FORMULA.

Do remember this: Your fat loss is correlated with your present body composition and diet. If, *like me*, you are already near your healthiest minimum body-fat composition and are eating a reasonably low-fat diet, your fat loss will necessarily be slower than those with more body fat. It may start out, as with me, at only half a pound (225 g) a week. Of course, I did not cut much below 60 grams of fat a day (aren't men lucky!). If you are a woman and wish to lose as quickly as possible, cut your fat intake to the bottom limit of the recommended range, that is, to 20 grams a day (men may cut to 30 grams a day).

Your ultimate guarantee of success in eliminating the final 5 to 15 pounds lies in making sure you include *fat-burning exercise* in your weight-management regimen. As I explain in Chapter Seven, many people are unaware that certain forms of exercise can make it very difficult to lose body fat and may even facilitate weight gain. If you are already an active person and losing those last few troublesome pounds has been truly difficult, the T-Factor Diet *and* the maximum fat-burning potential of the T-Factor Activity Programme are both essential.

WHAT OTHERS SAY ABOUT THE T-FACTOR DIET

In our own narratives, Ms Jamie Pope-Cordle and I tried to describe our experiences on the T-Factor Diet in ways that we hope will be helpful to you. Now I will report the experiences of other people who have used the diet with the same end in mind.

Ms K and her husband are employed by one of our local churches. She was more than 5 stone (34 kg) over recommended levels and Mr K was about 4 stone (25 kg) overweight when they began the programme under Jamie's guidance. I did not meet them until they had each lost about 3½ stone (23 kg). Mr K had been at his goal weight for several months, while his wife was still in the process of losing her last 20 pounds (9 kg).

When I asked what was different about this time, compared with other occasions when they had tried to lose weight, they both said, 'We were ready together. At other times it was just one of us, but this time we were ready to support each other and both do what it takes.'

I have always felt that it is very hard for one family member to make an effort to change her or his eating habits when no one else has an interest in doing so. And this is especially true of the wife and mother. I have seen it happen countless times. The woman announces her desire to begin a weight-management programme and the whole family responds 'You mean we have to go on a diet because *you're* trying to lose weight?' For some reason, this doesn't often happen to the man in the family! When he says he's going to lose some weight, the whole family tends to follow suit.

The nice thing about the T-Factor Diet is that it's a healthy diet for everyone. The basic diet, including all the menus and recipes, is suitable for the entire family. If you don't want to lose weight, just add more no-fat and low-fat foods. You can all do it together and be healthier even if you have no wish to be slimmer.*

I'm always interested in how people solve the three major problems associated with changing eating and activity habits:

1. What substitutes have they found for the high-fat foods they used to eat?

2. How do they manage to eat out and enjoy themselves?

3. What motivates them to continue, since there will always be some situations in which the temptation to return to old habits is very strong?

When Ms K began to diet, she was eating a daily average of 144 grams of fat, or 54 per cent of her 2,400 daily calories. Over 45 per cent of 3,000 daily calories, or 150 grams, in Mr K's diet were from fat sources. They ate many meals out at fast-food restaurants, and especially enjoyed Mexican and Italian dishes. Now, according to their latest eating records, their diet contains about 20 to 25 per cent fat calories. Ms K is remaining at under 40 grams per day and still losing weight, while Mr K is at approximately 50 grams per day and holding steady.

I asked about their levels of physical activity. Since I am such an advocate of activity, I was disappointed in their answers. But these answers are informative.

Mr K, who had been very active while losing weight, had dropped to 'one workout a week, but I do walk a lot every day in my job.' I suggested he get a pedometer and see just how far he really goes. Most people who think they move around a great deal don't move nearly as much as they think. I know: I move around as much as I can when I'm working, but it only adds up to about one mile per day. Mrs K had never become active at all. 'I'm just too busy to take the time, and I'd rather do it with my diet.'

Well, on the other hand, they are managing their weight very well by following the T-Factor Diet without becoming more active, which proves once again that the diet can be of help to sedentary people. But, on the other hand, I never feel very confident about the

* For people who do not wish to lose weight I suggest starting out by adding fat only to the top of the T-Factor ranges recommended for women and men, together with any amount of no-fat foods to satisfy the appetite. For most people this will result in an intake of about 20 per cent of total daily calories in fat. Recent research shows that while this may not lead to any appreciable weight loss in people who are already within the range of desirable weight it can lead to body composition changes. That is, people at desirable weight lose fat and replace it with lean tissues when they change the composition of their diets by replacing dietary fat with carbohydrate.

ability of anyone with tendencies to obesity to maintain a desirable weight without a daily activity programme. As I explain in Chapter Seven, physical activity helps to regulate appetite. Anyone who does not develop an active life-style will probably always feel a need for restraint, and that restraint can become oppressive.

When I asked the couple whether sticking to their programme ever presented any problems, Ms K said, 'Yes, sometimes. It doesn't happen very often, but we are both very busy. Our work requires that we eat out two-thirds of the time, and we are often pressed for time when we decide to cook at home. However, when we are tempted in a restaurant as the dessert tray comes around, we always split one dessert rather than each take one. And we have learned many new, quick, low-fat recipes for home cooking.'

When I asked what motivates them to adhere to the programme in spite of temptations, both of them responded enthusiastically about the change in the way they feel. 'I am down three dress sizes. I changed my hairdo. I switched from spectacles to contact lenses. When I meet people who haven't seen me for a year, they absolutely do not recognize me. I just like myself a whole lot better this way, and I'm not going to change.' Mr K echoed the exact same sentiments, adding, 'It's so much easier to move around now that I'm almost 60 pounds [4 stone/27 kg] lighter. I automatically take the stairs in our building, covering the three flights many times a day, and I walk wherever and whenever I can on business. I never try to conserve on the number of trips I need to make, as I used to.'

Although I am disappointed by their failure to increase and maintain an activity programme, I still think the couple will do well. They have started a T-Factor group in their church, and have been joined by members from another church. Perhaps the need to be good role models will reinforce their commitment. I think you, too, will find solid extra reinforcement for maintaining the T-Factor program if you recruit friends and co-workers to join you. There is great strength in social support. With all your friends helping you no one will sabotage your motivation to succeed.

COMMENTS FROM THE RESEARCH PARTICIPANTS IN THE VANDERBILT WEIGHT MANAGEMENT PROGRAM

During the past year we have been testing both versions of the T-Factor Diet at Vanderbilt. Half our research participants are in the no-calorie-cutting, no-calorie-counting group, and half use the

Quick Melt. Periodically we ask the participants to write comments and suggestions for their group leaders.

Here are the major comments that have been made by people who have followed the basic T-Factor Diet without trying to cut or count calories. They are distilled from the hundreds of weekly reports in our files.

The most frequent comment we receive is, first and foremost, 'I can't believe I'm eating like this and losing weight!' It's phrased in many different ways:

'It doesn't seem like a diet – I'm not counting calories!' AS

'I can't believe I can eat some of these high-calorie foods that are low in fat just as I desire, and lose weight.' JI

For many people who have resigned themselves to the idea that they must deprive themselves and periodically fight hunger in order to lose weight, it's an almost incredible experience. 'There is always something to eat *that tastes good* when I'm hungry.' CR

Here are some other comments in this vein:

'I have a large family, all working different shifts. I cook for all of them, and now I can nibble on no-fat foods and not feel like I'm starving myself.' FL

'I can eat bread! I'm not hungry.' DL

'I'm not hungry, yet I'm losing weight. Best – I'm changing my life-style.' JI

For those who have been a part of the calorie-counting diet culture all their lives the T-Factor Diet is a re-education in nutrition and the importance of reducing fat in the diet. Comments such as 'I didn't know where the fats are. I'm getting education in nutrition and exercise and there are nice tips on food' (VW) summarise this new awareness well.

Of course we want the T-Factor Diet to be effective in helping people who have had difficulty losing weight in other programmes, and it's nice to receive comments like this one, from someone who was on a 1,200-calorie diet in another programme and still could not lose weight: 'It works. I was in [a popular commercial programme] for two months before this and lost nothing. I'm thrilled!' JB.* Also 'I'm getting a consistent, gradual weight loss – my first success in years. It works!' RV

But naturally the most important issue is – *can you live with it?* Here are some quotes that address this important concern:

---

* On the commercial 1,200-calorie programme this woman was choosing foods that were high in fat. An analysis of her eating records showed over 50 per cent of calories from fat. She is now eating much more total food and far less fat, and is losing weight.

'This is a diet to live by, not three months on and then back to old eating habits.' ME

'It's great being able to eat at any time – all you want – so long as you watch the fat. It's wonderful for munchers like me.' AK

'The flexibility is a strong point. No rigid rules about substitutions and I'm learning the fat content of foods.' DL

'I was surprised to see how many good things there are that do not contain fat.' KD

'It's a life-style I can live with for the rest of my life. I never need to feel hungry or deprived. It's a logical, rational, good-health programme.' RF

Many people comment on the ease of implementing the diet:

'It is less time consuming that counting calories, and I don't feel like I'm dieting when I can eat sandwiches instead of cottage cheese all the time.' DL

'It's so easy. You absolutely don't feel deprived. It's not confusing.' JB

We want people to feel good. It's time to be done with obsessions and guilt over your eating habits. Our last comment shows that the diet does have the impact we desire on the digestive systems of people who have clogged themselves up with a high-fat diet:

'I feel better. I can see some increase in energy level. My friends say I look better, especially less tired. Psychologically, I feel better about myself since I'm taking care of myself as well as my family.' MS

CHAPTER FIVE

THE QUICK MELT AND THE TRANSITION TO MAINTENANCE

Having been 5 stone (34 kg) overweight myself I can certainly understand how you feel if you are eager to lose weight quickly. When I lost those 5 stone (34 kg) twenty-five years ago I used an alternating approach – three weeks of quick weight loss followed by a vacation period. I would repeat the quick-weight-loss diet whenever I felt motivated to do so, losing about a stone (7 kg) each time. I kept the weight off by becoming a tennis player and jogger, which helped me burn off whatever calories I chose to eat each day. Many years later my approach to losing weight evolved into the Rotation Diet. The T-Factor Quick Melt is an advance over the Rotation Diet but, like the Rotation Diet, it can be used to give people who want a quick weight loss the safe, fast results their desire.

Because I don't think it's wise from a psychological standpoint, or particularly good for your morale, to restrict food intake for long periods of time, I continue to recommend the appealing, time-limited, quick-weight-loss feature of the Rotation Diet in the T-Factor Quick Melt. Just as in the Rotation Diet, very overweight people may lose up to a pound (450 g) a day, and, depending on the number of optional snacks chosen (one is recommended), the average dieter will lose 9 to 12 pounds (4 to 5.5 kg) in three weeks.

HOWEVER, THE T-FACTOR QUICK MELT IS A SIGNIFICANT IMPROVEMENT OVER THE ROTATION DIET IN ONE KEY ASPECT – IT'S DESIGNED TO LEAD YOU ALONG THE ROUTE TO LASTING RESULTS RIGHT FROM DAY 1.

Here's why.

Although the Rotation Diet is a low-fat diet as well as a low-calorie diet *in its quick-loss phase*, it has, unfortunately, failed many people in maintenance. With its emphasis on calories, the Rotation Diet and its maintenance programme fail to stress the extreme importance of continuing to control fat intake at the level required for permanent weight control. That's because when I created the Rotation Diet, I was unaware of the direct relationship between the fat content of your body and the fat content of your diet. I want to stress this point once again: *The fat content of your body may be less related to your diet's total calories than it is to your daily fat intake.*

When you use the T-Factor Quick Melt, you will be following the basic fat-control principles of the T-Factor Diet. So, although you will be losing weight just about as quickly as with the Rotation Diet, you will still be learning, and, I hope, permanently adopting, the T-Factor fat-gram solution to your weight problem.

I think you will find the Quick Melt much easier and more comfortable to implement than other quick-loss plans because it not only permits you but *encourages* you to eat more of a larger variety of foods. *Unlike most other quick-loss plans, the T-Factor Quick Melt is a nutritious diet that meets the Recommended Dietary Allowances (RDAs) established by the United States National Research Council.*

The daily menus in this chapter each contain the fat levels I recommended in the T-Factor Diet – that is, 20 to 40 grams of fat per day for a woman and 30 to 60 grams for a man (see page 84 for adapting the menus for men). But, obviously, in order to lose weight even more quickly than you would on the basic T-Factor Diet, you have to cut calories. By cutting calories – not just substituting carbohydrates for fat – you create a deficit that pulls even more fat from your fat cells.

The daily menus in this chapter all contain approximately 1,000 calories for a woman, and 1,500 calories for a man. With an added snack (shown as optional on the menus) they will total between 1,100 and 1,300 calories per day for a woman and between 1,600 and 1,800 for a man.

Although there are twenty-one days of menus, you can repeat them over and over again as long as you wish. My personal preference is to take a break after three weeks of cutting calories, but the menus are nutritious enough (even at 1,000 calories for women and 1,500 for men) to be repeated for long periods of time. You can, occasionally, substitute one day's menu for another, one meal for another, or you can substitute different foods using the rules listed below. This variety will keep the diet interesting and lessen any feelings of deprivation you may have. However, don't eat the same meal or menu over and over again, to the virtual exclusion of other foods. The key to a healthy diet is to eat a wide variety of foods and not to slight any particular food group.

HOW FAST WILL YOU LOSE?

Weight loss on the Quick Melt is initially faster than on the basic T-Factor Diet because you are cutting calories and establishing a larger daily energy deficit. The deficit will at first be made up in part from your glycogen (carbohydrate) stores and in part from your fat stores. While the average participant in the Vanderbilt Weight Management Program who tested the Quick Melt and *added the daily snack* lost over 9 pounds (4 kg) in three weeks, people who are considerably overweight can begin with a weight loss of over a pound a day for a few days and end up losing as much as 21 pounds (10 kg) in twenty-one days.

If you are less than 3½ stone (23 kg) overweight, however, do not expect that rate of loss for more than a few days, or a week at most, for the following reasons.

As I explained in Chapter Two, when you cut calories, you burn part of your glycogen storage, as well as fat, in your fuel mixture. This causes an initial water loss. It occurs because only about 500 calories of glycogen are stored in a pound of the glycogen/water mixture in your liver and muscles (as compared to 3,500 calories in a pound of fat). Thus, for every 500 calories of glycogen loss, you lose a pound (450 g). In addition, the reduction in calories also means a reduction in sodium, which will increase your water losses.

On reduced calories you can lose several pounds in the first week before you reach a new equilibrium in glycogen storage and water balance. Your new level of glycogen storage will be somewhat lower than your normal standard. At this point your body will begin to draw upon its fat storage to a greater extent, using up more fat relative to glycogen, *and weight loss will slow considerably*. Since fat is stored at around 3,500 calories per pound (450 g) of fat tissue, compared with only 500 calories per pound of glycogen storage, weight loss may slow to about one-seventh the rate of your initial loss by the end of two or three weeks.

Weight loss in people who are not significantly overweight is also slower because they are not likely to be retaining so much water, and the calorie deficit created by the diet is less than for a severely overweight person. It only stands to reason that, other things being equal, a heavier person requires more calories to maintain his or her weight. An 18 stone (113 kg) person who cuts from an intake of 3,000 calories to 1,000 calories creates a deficit that's twice as large as that in an 11 stone (68 kg) person who cuts from 2,000 to 1,000. The heavier person will lose weight about twice as fast.

This slowdown in the rate of weight loss tends to be very discouraging. It will occur no matter what reduced-calorie diet you use. *So please understand how and why it occurs, and be assured that from the second or third week the losses will be entirely fat losses.*

Here is how you can calculate your expected average losses per week once you have established your new glycogen and water balance. Starting in Week 3, think in terms of those 3,500 calories per pound of fat. That is, you must have an energy deficit of 3,500 calories a week to lose a pound of fat per week. If your energy intake is approximately 1,000 calories less than your output each day, you will accumulate a deficit of about 7,000 calories per week and lose an average of about 2 pounds of fat weight per week. But, that's only 'on average'!

If you count calories while using the Quick Melt, remember that you will actually lose more true fat weight *by cutting fat calories* than by cutting carbohydrate calories. That's because fat is more available for use by the human body than carbohydrate. As I also explained in Chapter Two, 1,000 calories of fat has always provided you with more usable energy than 1,000 calories of carbohydrate, so your *actual* energy deficit will be greater than it might seem on paper if you cut fat calories rather from carbohydrates.

WEIGHT LOSS WILL NOT PROCEED LIKE CLOCKWORK.

Even if your caloric deficit averages 1,000 calories a day, you will not lose exactly 2 pounds (1 kg) per week. Sometimes you will gain! You will think your body is playing tricks on you, but it isn't. Cyclic hormonal changes can lead to several pounds of water retention. Stress can lead to weight gain. Under the severe stress accompanying the outbreak of war, for example, people have been known to gain several pounds overnight, due to water retention. Every salty pickle means a pound of water retention, and if you happen to use a salty dressing and also pickles it can mean 2 or 3 pounds. A Chinese dinner means 2 pounds (1 kg) for most people, including me, and 3 or 4 pounds for others who have stronger tendencies to retain water.

BUT IN SPITE OF THE SCALES' VARIATIONS THE FAT LOSS CONTINUES.

IS THERE ANY LIMIT TO THE TIME YOU CAN USE THE QUICK MELT?

There are a number of different ways to use the Quick Melt and you can suit your changing moods and inclinations.

Because the Quick Melt is designed to meet the RDAs and is well balanced and healthily low in fat, you can, if you like, stick with it until you lose all the weight you wish.

You can take a short break from dieting if you feel deprived, and you can continue to lose fat weight by following the T-Factor fat-gram formula. But, ADD CARBOHYDRATE CALORIES SLOWLY.

You can enter into a period of true maintenance BY ADDING CALORIES, INCLUDING BOTH CARBOHYDRATE *AND A LITTLE FAT*, VERY SLOWLY.

You must add calories slowly after a restricted-calorie diet in order to prevent water retention and a rapid weight gain. If you want to prevent water retention, be sure to read the final section of this chapter on making a transition to maintenance before increasing your intake after the Quick Melt.

HOW TO USE THE QUICK MELT MENUS

In contrast with the menus for the basic T-Factor Diet (Chapter Three) in which only the fatty foods are portion controlled, the menus here are entirely portion controlled. They are designed to contain between 1,100 and 1,300 calories per day for women and between 1,600 and 1,800 calories per day for men, including the snack. Your snack can be eaten at any time.

THE SUBSTITUTION RULE

Follow the menus as closely as you can, but if you don't like a particular selection, substitute *from within the same food group*. That is, you can substitute one vegetable for another, one fruit for another, one meat for another, etc. Try to keep to similar foods – a green for a green, a citrus fruit for a citrus – when you can. That's because we want you to preserve the spectrum of nutrients as much as possible. You may also settle on three or four favourite breakfasts and lunches, and rotate among them, but keep in mind that a wide variety of different foods helps ensure sound nutrition.

DO YOU NEED VITAMIN AND MINERAL SUPPLEMENTS?

When you reduce calories there is always the danger that you will be a bit deficient in one or another vitamin or mineral if you stick with that reduction for a long period of time, that is, more than three weeks. The wide variety of foods in the menus below helps ensure that you will meet the Recommended Dietary Allowances and obtain sound nutrition, but if you substitute and limit variety beyond my recommendations, I suggest you take a multiple vitamin and mineral tablet that contains from 100 to 150 per cent of the RDAs for the key nutrients. DO NOT TAKE MEGADOSES OF VITAMINS EXCEPT FOR SOME SPECIFIC MEDICAL PURPOSE, AND THEN ONLY UNDER THE GUIDANCE OF A KNOWLEDGEABLE PHYSICIAN.

T-FACTOR QUICK MELT MENUS

WEEK 1

[DAY 1]

Breakfast ½ banana; 1 oz/28 g of dry cereal (1 g); 8 fl oz/ 225 ml skimmed milk or ½ skimmed/½ semi-skimmed (0–2 g); coffee or tea
  Total fat: 1–3 g

Lunch 2 oz/56 g of water-packed tuna (1 g); 1 scant teaspoon of mayonnaise (4 g); 1 small roll (1 g); alfalfa sprouts and assorted raw vegetables; 1 apple; no-cal beverage
  Total fat: 6 g

Dinner 3 oz/80 g of lean beef (12 g); 1 medium baked potato; 2 small courgettes; large tossed salad no- or low-cal salad dressing (2 dessertspoons = 0–3 g); no-call beverage
  Total fat: 12–15 g

Snack 8 fl oz/225 ml very low fat plain yoghurt; 4 oz/ 110 g unsugared strawberries; 3 rice cakes (1 g)
  Total fat: 1 g
  Total fat for Day 1: 20–25 g

73

[DAY 2]

Breakfast   ½ grapefruit; 1 roll or 2 crumpets (2 g); 2 scant teaspoons jam or marmalade; 8 fl oz/225 ml skimmed milk or ½ skimmed/½ low fat (0–2 g); coffee or tea

Total fat: 2–4 g

Lunch   2 oz/156 g of turkey (2 g); ½ 6 inch/15 cm pitta pocket (1 g); sliced tomato; assorted raw vegetables; mustard; no- or low-cal salad dressing (2 dessertspoons = 0–3 g); 1 pear; no-cal beverage

Total fat: 3–6 g

Dinner   4½ oz/125 g of baked or grilled fish (4 g); 3 rounded tablespoons of brown or wild rice (1 g); 1 serving of steamed broccoli; 1 serving of carrots; 1 piece fresh fruit; no-cal beverage

Total fat: 5 g

Snack   3 rice cakes (1 g), 2 pieces fresh fruit

Total fat: 1 g

Total fat for Day 2: 11–16 g

[DAY 3]

Breakfast   3 rounded tablespoons blackberries or other seasonal fruit; 1 oz/28 g of dry cereal (1 g); 8 fl oz/225 ml skimmed milk or ½ skimmed/½ semi-skimmed milk (0–2 g); coffee or tea

Total fat: 1–3 g

Lunch   Cheese toast: 1 oz/28 g cheese (8–10 g); 1 slice of wholegrain bread (1 g); 8 fl oz/225 ml Gazpacho or consommé (see recipe section; 0–2 g); 1 orange; no-cal beverage

Total fat: 9–13 g

Dinner   3½ oz/100 g chicken (3.5 g); 3–4 boiled new potatoes; 1 serving french or runner beans; large tossed salad; no- or low-cal salad dressing (2 dessertspoons = 0–3 g); 1 apple, no-cal beverage

Total fat: 3½–6½ g

Snack   8 fl oz/225 ml very low fat plain yoghurt; ½ banana; 3 rice cakes (1 g)

Total fat: 1 g

Total fat for Day 3: 14½–22½

Breakfast   2 rounded tablespoons porridge or other hot cereal (1 g); 2 dessertspoons of raisins; 8 fl oz/225 ml skimmed milk or ½ skimmed/½ semi-skimmed (0–2 g); 1 slice of wholegrain bread (1 g); coffee or tea
> *Total fat: 2–4 g*

Lunch   2 oz/56 g of leftover chicken for sandwich (2 g); 1 wholewheat roll (2 g); tomato slices, lettuce leaves; 1 scant teaspoon of mayonnaise (4 g); 3 rounded tablespoons unsugared pineapple chunks; no-cal beverage
> *Total fat: 8 g*

Dinner   1 serving of Pork Tenderloin with Orange Marmalade (page 124; 3 g); 1 serving of cauliflower; 3 tablespoons of unsweetened apple sauce; large tossed salad; no- or low-cal salad dressing (2 dessertspoons = 0–3 g); 1 Massachusetts Corn Muffin (page 95; 3 g); no-cal beverage
> *Total fat: 6–9 g*

Snack   1 oz/28 g of dry cereal (1 g); 3 tablespoons unsugared sliced peaches; 8 fl oz/225 ml skimmed milk or ½ skimmed/½ semi-skimmed (0–2 g)
> *Total fat: 1–3 g*   *Total fat for Day 4: 17–24 g*

Breakfast   Large slice honeydew melon or 2 pieces other seasonal fruit; 1 egg, poached (5 g); 1 slice of wholegrain toast (1 g); 8 fl oz/225 ml skimmed milk (0–2 g); coffee or tea
> *Total fat: 6–8 g*

Lunch   8 fl oz/225 ml bouillon-based, vegetable soup (2 g); 2 tablespoons croutons (1 g); chef's salad: 16 fl oz/450 ml measure of assorted raw vegetables, 1 oz/28 g turkey (1 g); ½ oz/14 g cheese (4–5 g); no- or low-cal salad dressing (2 dessertspoons = 0–3 g); 1 piece fresh fruit; no-cal beverage
> *Total fat: 8–12 g*

Dinner   1 serving of Picadillo and Cornbread Wedges (page 134; 9 g); large tossed salad; no- or low-cal salad dressing (2 dessertspoons = 0–3 g); 1 apple; no-cal beverage
> *Total fat: 9–12 g*

Snack   3 rice cakes (1 g), 2 pieces fresh fruit
> *Total fat: 1 g*   *Total fat for Day 5: 24–33 g*

[DAY 6]

Breakfast   3 rounded tablespoons sliced fruit; 1 oz/28 g dry cereal (1 g); 8 fl oz/225 ml skimmed milk or ½ skimmed/½ semi-skimmed (0–2 g); coffee or tea
Total fat: 1–3 g

Lunch   2 oz/56 g tinned salmon (4 g); 5 Ryvita (1 g); assorted raw vegetables; no- or low-cal salad dressing (2 dessertspoons = 0–3 g); 1 orange; no-cal beverage
Total fat: 5–8 g

Dinner   3½ oz/100 g chicken breast (3.5 g); 1 serving Brussels sprouts or other green vegetable; 1 serving of Scalloped Potatoes (page 144; 3.5 g); large tossed salad; no- or low-cal salad dressing (2 dessertspoons = 0–3 g); 1 slice of wholegrain bread (1 g); no-cal beverage
Total fat: 8–11 g

Snack   8 fl oz/225 ml very low fat plain yoghurt; 2 dessertspoons of sultanas; 3 rice cakes (1 g)
Total fat: 1 g
Total fat for Day 6: 15–23 g

[DAY 7]

Breakfast   ½ grapefruit; 1 roll (1 g); 2 scant teaspoons of jam or marmalade; 8 fl oz/225 ml skimmed milk or ½ skimmed/½ low fat (0–2 g); coffee or tea
Total fat: 1–3 g

Lunch   4 oz/110 g of low-fat cottage cheese (3 g); 2–3 pieces assorted fresh fruit; 1 home-made muffin (see page 94; 3 g); assorted raw vegetables; no-cal beverage
Total fat: 6 g

Dinner   1 serving Quick Turkey Chop Suey (page 130; 8 g); 3 rounded tablespoons of brown rice (1 g); large tossed salad; no- or low-cal salad dressing (2 dessertspoons = 0–3 g); 1 slice of wholegrain bread (1 g); no-cal beverage
Total fat: 10–13 g

Snack   1 oz/28 g of dry cereal (1 g); ½ banana; 8 fl oz/225 ml skimmed milk or ½ skimmed/½ semi-skimmed (0.2 g)
Total fat: 1–3 g
Total fat for Day 7: 18–25 g

WEEK 2

[DAY 8]

Breakfast   ½ grapefruit; 1 roll (1 g); 2 scant teaspoons of jam or marmalade; 8 fl oz/225 ml skimmed milk or ½ skimmed/½ low fat (0–2 g); coffee or tea
Total fat: 1–3 g

Lunch   2 oz/56 g of sliced turkey (2 g); 2 slices of whole-grain bread (2 g); sliced tomato; lettuce leaves; assorted raw vegetables; 1 apple; no-cal beverage
Total fat: 4 g

Dinner   1 serving Pasta and Shrimp with Ricotta Cheese Sauce (page 137; 7 g); 1 serving french or runner beans; large tossed salad; no- or low-cal salad dressing (2 dessertspoons = 0–3 g); 1 piece fresh fruit; no-cal beverage
Total fat: 7–10 g

Snack   3 rice cakes (1 g), 3 tablespoons Fruit Topping or Meat Spread (pages 92, 99; 0–0.5 g)
Total fat: 2 g
Total fat for Day 8: 14–19 g

[DAY 9]

Breakfast   1 piece fresh fruit; 1 oz/28 g of dry cereal (1 g); 8 fl oz/225 ml skimmed milk or ½ skimmed/½ semi-skimmed (0-2 g); coffee or tea
Total fat: 1–3 g

Lunch   2 oz /56 g of water-packed tuna (1 g); 3 stalks celery, onion rings; sliced tomato; lettuce leaves; 1 scant teaspoon of mayonnaise (4 g); 2 slices of whole-grain bread (2 g); 1 orange; no-cal beverage
Total fat: 7 g

Dinner   1 serving of Aubergine Parmesan (page 133; 8 g); 3 rounded tablespoons cooked pasta (2 g); large tossed salad; no- or low-cal salad dressing (2 dessertspoons = 0–3 g); small bunch seedless grapes; no-cal beverage
Total fat: 10–13 g

Snack   8 fl oz/225 ml very low fat plain yoghurt; ½ banana; 5 Ryvita (1 g)
Total fat: 1 g
Total fat for Day 9: 19–24 g

Breakfast   3 rounded tablespoons porridge or other hot cereal (1 g); 2 dessertspoons of raisins; 8 fl oz/225 ml skimmed milk or ½ skimmed/½ semi-skimmed (0–2 g); 1 slice of wholegrain toast (1 g); coffee or tea
Total fat: 2–4 g

Lunch   Cheese toast: 1 oz/28 g of cheese (8–10 g), 1 slice of whole-grain bread (1 g); 8 fl oz/225 ml Corn Chowder or Minestrone (pages 107, 108; 1–2 g); 1 apple; no-cal beverage
Total fat: 10–13 g

Dinner   3½ oz/100 g of baked or grilled chicken (3.5 g); 1 serving of Apple-Sweet Sweet Potatoes (page 141, 1 g); 1 serving broccoli; large tossed salad; no- or low-cal salad dressing (2 dessertspoons = 0–3 g); no-cal beverage
Total fat: 4½–7½ g

Snack   1 oz/28 g of dry cereal (1 g); 8 fl oz/225 ml skimmed milk or ½ skimmed/½ semi-skimmed (0–2 g); 3 rounded tablespoons unsugared peach slices or other seasonal fruit
Total fat: 1–3 g
Total fat for Day 10: 17½–27½ g

Breakfast   ½ grapefruit; 1 egg, cooked without fat (5 g); 1 slice of whole-grain toast (1 g); 8 fl oz/225 ml skimmed milk or ½ skimmed/½ low fat (0–2 g); coffee or tea
Total fat: 6–8 g

Lunch   2 oz/56 g of leftover chicken (2 g); ½ 6 inch/15 cm pitta pocket (1 g); assorted raw vegetables; 1 piece seasonal fruit; no-cal beverage
Total fat: 3 g

Dinner   1 serving of Saucy Pastitiso (page 120; 10 g); large tossed salad; no- or low-cal salad dressing (2 dessertspoons = 0–3 g); 1 pear; no-cal beverage
Total fat: 10–13 g

Snack   5 Ryvita (1 g); 2 oz/56 g herb-flavoured low-fat cottage cheese (1 g)
Total fat: 2 g
Total fat for Day 11: 21–26 g

Breakfast   ½ banana; 1 oz/28 g of dry cereal (1 g); 8 fl oz/225 ml skimmed milk or ½ skimmed/½ semi-skimmed (0–2 g); coffee or tea

  Total fat: 1–3 g

Lunch   Spinach salad: 4–6 oz/110–175 g) spinach; 2 oz/56 g sliced fresh mushrooms; ½ hard-boiled egg (3 g); ½ oz/14 g of part-skim white cheese (4 g); 2 tablespoons chopped onions; 2 tablespoons croutons (1 g); no- or low-cal salad dressing (2 dessertspoons = 0–3 g); 1 slice of whole-grain bread (1 g); 1 peach; no-cal beverage

  Total fat: 9–12 g

Dinner   1 serving of Basic Better Beans (page 131; 5 g); 3 rounded tablespoons brown rice (1 g); 1 serving Courgette Mushroom Mix (page 145; 1.5 g); 1 Massachusetts Corn Muffin (page 95; 3 g); large tossed salad; no- or low-cal salad dressing (2 dessertspoons = 0–3 g); 1 piece sliced fresh fruit; no-cal beverage

  Total fat: 10½–13½ g

Snack   8 fl oz/225 ml very low fat plain yoghurt; 2 dessertspoons of raisins; 3 rice cakes (1 g)

  Total fat: 1 g   *Total fat for Day 12: 21½–29½ g*

Breakfast   3 rounded tablespoons raspberries or other fruit; 1 oz/28 g dry cereal (1 g); 8 fl oz/225 ml skimmed milk or ½ skimmed/½ semi-skimmed (0–2 g); coffee or tea

  Total fat: 1–3 g

Lunch   8 fl oz/225 ml low-fat bought or home-made soup (2 g); 1 roll (1 g); ½ oz/14 g of part-skimmed ricotta or other cheese (5 g); assorted raw vegetables; 1 orange; no-cal beverage

  Total fat: 8 g

Dinner   1 pattie Salmon Croquettes Béarnaise (5½ g); 1 medium baked potato (or 1 serving of Scandinavian-Style Potato Casserole, page 144; 4.5 g); 1 serving French or runner beans; large tossed salad; no- or low-cal salad dressing (2 dessertspoons = 0–3 g); 1 slice of whole-grain bread (1 g); 1 nectarine or other fruit; no-cal beverage

  Total fat: 6–13½ g

Snack   5 Ryvita (1 g); 3 tablespoons Fruit Topping or Crabmeat Spread (pages 92, 99; 0.05 g)

  Total fat: 2 g   *Total fat for Day 13: 16–26½ g*

[DAY 14]
Breakfast   ½ grapefruit; 2 crumpets (2 g); 2 scant teaspoons
               of jam or marmalade; 8 fl oz/225 ml skimmed milk
               or ½ skimmed/½ low fat (0–2 g); coffee or tea
                    Total fat: 2–4 g

Lunch   4 oz/110 g of low-fat cottage cheese (3 g); 4 table-
               spoons assorted sliced fresh fruit; assorted raw
               vegetables; 1 home-made muffin (3 g); no-cal
               beverage
                    Total fat: 6 g

Dinner   3½ oz/100 g of baked or grilled chicken (3.5 g); 1
               serving of broccoli; 3 rounded tablespoons brown
               or wild rice (1 g); large tossed salad; no- or low-cal
               salad dressing (2 dessertspoons = 0–3 g); 1 slice
               melon; no-cal beverage
                    Total fat: 4½–7½ g

Snack   1 oz/28 g of dry cereal (1 g); 3 rounded table-
               spoons unsugared raspberries; 8 fl oz/225 ml skim-
               med milk or ½ skimmed/½ semi-skimmed (0–2 g)
                    Total fat: 1–3 g
                    Total fat for Day 14: 13½–20½ g

WEEK 3

[DAY 15]
Breakfast   1 piece fruit in season; 1 roll or 2 crumpets (2 g);
               2 scant teaspoons of jam or marmalade; 8 fl oz/
               225 ml skimmed milk or ½ skimmed/½ low fat
               (0–2 g); coffee or tea
                    Total fat: 2–4 g

Lunch   Stuffed tomato: 1 whole tomato, 2 oz/56 g of
               water-packed tuna (1 g); assorted raw vegetables,
               no- or low-cal salad dressing (2 dessertspoons =
               0–3 g); 5 Ryvita (1 g); small bunch seedless
               grapes; no-cal beverage
                    Total fat: 2–5 g

Dinner   3 oz/85 g of lean beefsteak (see page 116; 7.5 g); 1
               medium baked potato; 1 serving cooked spinach;
               1 slice of whole-grain bread (1 g); 1 apple; no-cal
               beverage
                    Total fat: 8½ g

Snack   3 rice cakes (1 g); 2 pieces fresh fruit
                    Total fat: 1 g
                    Total fat for Day 15: 13½–18½ g

Breakfast 3 rounded tablespoons peach slices or seasonal fruit; 1 oz/28 g of dry cereal (1 g); 8 fl oz/225 ml skimmed milk or ½ skimmed/½ semi-skimmed (0–2 g); coffee or tea
Total fat: 1–3 g

Lunch Toasted pitta pocket: 1 oz/28 g of cheese (8–10 g), ½ 6-inch/15 cm wholegrain pitta (1 g); sliced tomato; alfalfa sprouts, and other vegetables of choice; 1 orange; no-cal beverage
Total fat: 9–11 g

Dinner 4½ oz/125 g of baked or grilled fish (4 g); 3 rounded tablespoons spinach noodles or other pasta (1 g); 1 serving Beetroot a l'Orange (page 142); large tossed salad; no- or low-cal salad dressing (2 dessertspoons = 0–3 g); 3 rounded tablespoons pineapple chunks; no-cal beverage
Total fat: 5–8 g

Snack 8 fl oz/225 ml very low fat plain yoghurt; ½ banana; 3 rice cakes (1 g)
Total fat: 1 g
Total fat for Day 16: 16–24 g

[DAY 17]

Breakfast 1 serving melon; 1 egg, cooked without fat (5 g); 1 slice of whole-grain toast (1 g); 8 fl oz/225 ml skimmed milk or ½ skimmed/½ low fat (0–2 g); coffee or tea
Total fat: 6–8 g

Lunch Chef's salad: large salad of assorted raw vegetables, 1 oz/28 g of turkey (1 g); ½ oz/14 g of shredded hard cheese (4–5 g); 2 tablespoons croutons (1 g), no- or low-cal salad dressing (2 dessertspoons = 0–3 g); 1 home-made muffin (3 g); no-cal beverage
Total fat: 9–13 g

Dinner 1 serving Spinach Lasagne (page 135; 8–10 g); green salad; no- or low-cal salad dressing (2 dessertspoons = 0–3 g); no-cal beverage
Total fat: 8–13 g

Snack 1 oz/28 g of dry cereal (1 g); 1 piece fruit, sliced; 8 fl oz/225 ml skimmed milk (0–2 g)
Total fat: 1 g
Total fat for Day 17: 24–35 g

Breakfast 3 rounded tablespoons porridge or other hot cereal (1 g); 2 dessertspoons of sultanas; 8 fl oz/ 225 ml skimmed milk or ½ skimmed/½ semi-skimmed (0–2 g); 1 slice of whole-grain toast (1 g); coffee or tea
> *Total fat: 2–4 g*

Lunch 1 serving Corn Chowder (page 107; 2 g); 1 roll (2 g); 2 oz/56 g part-skimmed ricotta cheese (4–5 g); assorted raw vegetables; 1 apple; no-cal beverage.
> *Total fat: 8–9 g*

Dinner 3½ oz/100 g of baked or grilled chicken (3.5 g); 1 medium baked potato; 1 serving Brussels sprouts or other green vegetable; large tossed salad; no- or low-cal salad dressing (2 dessertspoons = 0–3 g); 1 piece fresh fruit; no-cal beverage
> *Total fat: 3½–6½ g*

Snack 5 Ryvita (1 g); 3 tablespoons Fruit Topping or Meat Spread (0–½ g)
> *Total fat: 2 g*
> *Total fat for Day 18: 14½–20½ g*

[DAY 19]

Breakfast 1 piece fruit, sliced; 1 oz/28 g of dry cereal (1 g) 8 fl oz/225 ml skimmed milk or ½ skimmed/½ semi-skimmed (0–2 g); coffee or tea
> *Total fat: 1–3 g*

Lunch 2 oz/56 g of leftover chicken breast (2 g); 2 slices of whole-grain bread (2 g); lettuce; tomato slices; 1 scant teaspoon of mayonnaise (4 g); 1 slice watermelon or other fruit in season; no-cal beverage
> *Total fat: 8 g*

Dinner 1 serving of Pork Tenderloin with Orange Marmalade (page 124; 3 g); 3 rounded tablespoons peas; 1 serving cauliflower; large tossed salad; no- or low-cal salad dressing (2 dessertspoons = 0–3 g); 1 slice of whole-grain bread (1 g); 1 apple; no-cal beverage
> *Total fat: 4–7 g*

Snack 8 fl oz/225 ml very low fat plain yoghurt; 4 oz/110 g unsugared strawberries; 3 rice cakes (1 g)
> *Total fat: 1 g*
> *Total fat for Day 19: 14–19 g*

[DAY 20]

Breakfast
½ grapefruit; 1 roll or 2 crumpets (2 g); 2 scant teaspoons jam or marmalade; 8 fl oz/225 ml skimmed milk or ½ skimmed/½ low fat (0–2 g); coffee or tea
Total fat: 2–4 g

Lunch
4 oz/110 g low-fat cottage cheese (3 g); 3 rounded tablespoons unsugared sliced fruit; 1 home-made muffin (3 g); assorted raw vegetables; no-cal beverage
Total fat: 6 g

Dinner
4½ oz/125 g of baked or grilled fish (4 g); 3 rounded tablespoons brown or wild rice (1 g); 1 serving French or runner beans; large tossed salad; no- or low-cal salad dressing (2 dessertspoons = 0–3 g); 1 whole-grain roll (2 g); 1 pear; no-cal beverage
Total fat: 7–10 g

Snack
1 oz/28 g of dry cereal (1 g); ½ banana; 8 fl oz/225 ml skimmed milk or ½ skimmed/½ semi-skimmed (0–2 g)
Total fat: 1–3 g   *Total fat for Day 20: 16–23 g*

[DAY 21]

Breakfast
3 rounded tablespoons unsugared berries or sliced fruit; 1 oz/28 g cereal (1 g); 8 fl oz/225 ml skimmed milk or ½ skimmed/½ semi-skimmed (0–2 g); coffee or tea
Total fat: 1–3 g

Lunch
2 oz/56 g of sliced turkey (2 g); 2 slices of whole-grain bread (2 g); sliced tomato; alfalfa sprouts; assorted raw vegetables; 1 orange; no-cal beverage
Total fat: 4 g

Dinner
3½ oz/98 g of baked or grilled chicken (3½ g); 3 rounded tablespoons broad beans; 2 small courgettes; large tossed salad; no- or low-cal salad dressing (2 dessertspoons = 0–3 g); 1 slice of whole-grain bread (1 g); 1 piece fresh fruit; no-cal beverage
Total fat: 4½–7½ g

Snack
5 Ryvita (1 g); 2 oz/56 g seasoned low-fat cottage cheese (1.5 g)
Total fat: 2 g   *Total fat for Day 21: 11½–16½ g*

83

ADAPTING THE QUICK MELT MENUS FOR MEN

The male version of the Quick Melt calls for 1,600–1,800 calories per day and a fat-gram range of 30–60 grams. This level is easily obtained by increasing the portion sizes of the main dishes in the above menus, as well as the starchy side dishes, by 50 per cent. In addition, men may have two extra slices of bread each day. By adjusting portions in this way, everyone in the family can eat the same dishes and there is no need to prepare any special foods.

THE TRANSITION TO MAINTENANCE

WHY SHOULD YOU ADD CALORIES AND CARBO-HYDRATES SLOWLY AFTER A RESTRICTED DIET?

After an increase in total calories, or even in exclusively carbohydrate foods, there is a quick rehydration effect. On reduced calories, your body has been at a low point in glycogen storage and water balance. If you add calories quickly, it's as though your body has been lying in wait for this very opportunity. Your depleted glycogen stores go up about a pound in weight for every increase of 500 calories of glycogen stored. There is also an increase in body fluid due to the additional sodium that occurs naturally in many foods. The carbohydrate itself stimulates a temporary increase in water retention throughout the system. Taken together, your body may even overshoot its normal water balance and take a few days to return to a lower equilibrium.

If you add calories and carbohydrates slowly, you can continue to lose body fat while you slowly rehydrate. For example, if you gradually go up to a maintenance level over a one-week period, you can continue to lose enough additional body fat to equal the increase in body fluid. Only in this way can you come out even on the scales.*

Daily exercise will also help to prevent water retention. Water will be lost through perspiration. In addition, your breath is 100 per cent saturated with moisture, so any increase in breathing rate due to exercise means more water lost.

Remember to drink plenty of water; it helps to stimulate kidney action. Of course, avoid foods high in sodium and increase your intake of fruits and vegetables, which are high in potassium. A high potassium to sodium ratio in your diet helps to prevent water retention.

When you finish the transition, begin to use the fat-gram-

---

* A complete explanation of how the body stabilizes at a new weight and fat content is given in Appendix A.

controlled menus in the basic T-Factor Diet that are found in Chapter Three. If you have not already reached a low point in your body-fat content you will continue to lose additional weight without attempting to cut or count calories. Keep your fat-gram count in the recommended daily range of 20 to 40 grams for women and 30 to 60 grams for men. Add non-fatty foods in larger portions to your meals and use them as snacks until you reach a new equilibrium in your weight. Only experience can tell just what this weight will be, but remember that you will keep lost weight off for ever so long as you stick with a low-fat diet and satisfy your appetite with complex-carbohydrate foods.

TRANSITION MENUS

The first three days of the following menus contain between 1,400 and 1,500 calories. The last four days contain between 1,600 and 1,800 calories. The fat-gram count each day is low enough for you to add a scant teaspoon of extra fat or oil, as a spread or for cooking, and still not exceed the recommended level.

Men may increase portion sizes of main courses and side dishes by 50 per cent and add two extra slices of whole-grain bread or its equivalent each day.

[DAY 1]

Breakfast	1 serving of fresh fruit of choice; 8 fl oz/225 ml hot cereal (2 g); 2 dessertspoons raisins; 8 fl oz/225 ml skimmed milk (or ½ skimmed/½ low fat) (0–2 g); coffee or tea *Total fat: 2–4 g*
Lunch	Spinach salad: 8 oz/225 g fresh spinach; 2 oz/56 g sliced fresh mushrooms; 1 hard-boiled egg (5 g); 1 dessertspoon of grated cheese (4 g); 2 slices mild onion, no- or low-cal salad dressing (2 dessertspoons = 0–3 g); choice of muffin (3 g); 1 orange; no-cal beverage *Total fat: 12–15 g*
Dinner	4 oz/112 g Baked Chicken with Tarragon and Fennel or Light and Easy Lemon Chicken (4 g); 1 helping steamed broccoli; 3 rounded tablespoons cooked brown or wild rice (1 g); 1 serving of Elegant Pears (page 156; 2 g); no-cal beverage *Total fat: 7 g*
Snack	3 rice cakes (1 g); 1 piece fresh fruit *Total fat: 1 g* *Total fat for Day 1: 22–27 g*

[DAY 2]

Breakfast
1 oz/28 g of dry cereal (1 g); 1 banana; 8 fl oz/ 225 ml skimmed or low-fat milk (0–2 g); coffee or tea
Total fat: 1–3 g

Lunch
6 oz/175 g low-fat cottage cheese (4.5 g); choice of muffin (3 g) or serving of crispbreads (1–2 g); assorted raw vegetables: ½ sliced melon; no-cal beverage
Total fat: 8½–9½ g

Dinner
1 serving of Shrimps Florentine (page 113; 7 g) or 4 oz/110 g of baked, steamed or grilled fish; 1 serving of cooked French or runner beans; 1 medium baked potato; 1 slice of whole-grain bread (1 g); 1 apple; no-cal beverage
Total fat: 8 g

Snack
8 fl oz/225 ml very low fat plain yoghurt; 1 piece fresh fruit; 2 crispbreads (1 g)
Total fat: 1 g
Total fat for Day 2: 18½–21½ g

[DAY 3]

Breakfast
2 Oatmeal Pancakes (page 93; 4 g); 8 fl oz/225 ml skimmed or low-fat milk (0–2 g); 1 serving of fresh fruit of choice; coffee or tea
Total fat: 4–6 g

Lunch
8 fl oz/225 ml home-made soup of choice (2 g); turkey sandwich: 2 slices of whole-grain bread (2 g), 1 oz/28 g of turkey breast (1 g); sliced tomato, lettuce, beansprouts, 1 scant teaspoon of mayonnaise (4 g); 1 orange; no-cal beverage
Total fat: 9 g

Dinner
1 serving of Spinach Lasagne (page 135; 8 g) or Aubergine Parmesan (page 133; 8 g) (add 4 oz/ 110 g cooked pasta (2 g) with Aubergine Parmesan); 1 whole-grain roll (2 g); large tossed salad; no- or low-cal salad dressing (2 dessertspoons = 0–3 g); 1 serving of fresh fruit; no-cal beverage
Total fat: 10–13 g

Snack
1 oz/28 g dry cereal (1 g); 8 fl oz/225 ml skimmed or low-fat milk (0–2 g); 1 banana
Total fat: 1–3 g
Total fat for Day 3: 24–33 g

Breakfast ½ honeydew melon or other seasonal fruit; 1 egg, cooked without fat (5 g); 2 slices of whole-grain bread (2 g); 8 fl oz/225 ml skimmed milk or ½ skimmed/½ low fat (0–2 g)
Total fat: 7–9 g

Lunch Tuna-stuffed tomato: 2-3 oz/56-80 g of water-packed tuna (1 g), 1 scant teaspoon of mayonnaise (4 g), chopped celery, large whole tomato; 5 Ryvita (1 g); 1 orange; no-cal beverage
Total fat: 6 g

Dinner 1 serving of Swedish Meatballs (page 121; 14 g); 3 rounded tablespoons brown or wild rice (1 g); 1 serving steamed broccoli; large tossed salad; no- or low-cal salad dressing (2 dessertspoons = 0–3 g); fresh fruit; no-cal beverage
Total fat: 15–18 g

Snack 3 rice cakes (1 g); small helping of dried fruit
Total fat: 1 g   *Total fat for Day 4: 29–34 g*

[DAY 5]
Breakfast ½ grapefruit (or choice of fruit); 1 wholemeal bap (2 g); 2 scant teaspoons of preserves; 8 fl oz/225 ml skimmed milk or ½ skimmed/½ low fat (0–2 g); coffee or tea
Total fat: 2–4 g

Lunch 8 fl oz/225 ml Minestrone (page 108; 1 g); tuna salad sandwich: 2 slices of whole-wheat bread (2 g), 2–3 oz/56–80 g of water-packed tuna (1 g), chopped celery, ½ oz/14 g chopped green olives (about 4 medium, 2 g), 1 scant teaspoon of mayonnaise (4 g), sliced tomato, lettuce; 1 apple; no-cal beverage
Total fat: 10 g

Dinner 1 serving Indian Spiced Beans (page 133; 1 g); 3 rounded tablespoons brown rice (1 g); 2 dessertspoons grated cheese (9 g); Salsa (page 104); choice of chopped raw vegetables (e.g., lettuce, spring onions, green peppers, tomatoes); 1 serving of Lemon Meringue Pie (page 157; 5½ g); no-cal beverage
Total fat: 16½ g

Snack Choice of 1 serving of fresh or dried fruit
Total fat: 0   *Total fat for Day 5: 28½–30½ g*

Breakfast   1 oz/28 g dry cereal (1 g); sliced peaches (or choice of fruit for cereal); 8 fl oz/225 ml skimmed or low-fat milk (0–2 g); 1 slice of whole-wheat bread (1 g); 1 scant teaspoon of preserves; coffee or tea
Total fat: 2–4 g

Lunch   2 oz/56 g of turkey or chicken (2 g); ½ toasted pitta pocket (1 g); sliced tomato; assorted raw vegetables; mustard; no- or low-cal salad dressing (2 dessertspoons = 0–3 g); 1 pear (or choice of fruit); no-cal beverage
Total fat: 3–6 g

Dinner   1 serving Royal Indian Salmon (page 111; 10 g); small serving green peas; 3 rounded table-spoons brown or wild rice (1 g); large tossed salad; no- or low-cal salad dressing (2 dessertspoons = 0–3 g); 1 serving Poppy-Seed Cake (page 158; 7 g); no-cal beverage
Total fat: 18–21 g

Snack   1 cup of very low fat plain yoghurt; 1 banana; 3 rice cakes (1 g)
Total fat: 1 g   *Total fat for Day 6: 24–32 g*

[DAY 7]

Breakfast   1 serving of porridge or other hot cereal (2 g); 2 dessertspoons sultanas; 8 fl oz/225 ml skimmed or low-fat milk (0–2 g); 1 slice of whole-grain toast (1 g); 1 scant teaspoon honey; 1 piece fresh fruit; coffee or tea
Total fat: 3–5 g

Lunch   8 fl oz/225 ml home-made soup (2 g); 1 tablespoon croutons (2 g); chef's salad; assorted raw vege-tables; 1 oz/28 g turkey (1 g); ½ oz/14 g cheese (4–5 g); no- or low-cal salad dressing (2 des-sertspoons = 0–3 g); 1 apple; no-cal beverage
Total fat: 8–12 g

Dinner   4½ oz/125 g of Round-Roast Oriental (page 119; 13–14 g) or same quantity lean beefsteak; 1 medium baked potato; 1 serving Brussels Sprouts with Cara-way Seeds (page 143; 1 g) or other green vegetable; 1 hard wholewheat roll (2 g) 1 serving of Cocoa Pud-ding Cake (page 156; 4 g) or other T-Factor dessert recipe of your choice; no-cal beverage
Total fat: 20–21 g

Snack   1 serving of fresh or dried fruit
                    Total fat: 0
                    Total fat for Day 7: 31–38 g

CHAPTER SIX

RECIPES

INTRODUCTION

All the recipes in this chapter have been tested and tasted repeatedly by members of my family, friends and nutritionists at the Vanderbilt Weight Management Program and in the *Family Circle* test kitchen. They are delicious.

Most can be prepared in 10 to 20 minutes (not including cooking time), though there are a few 'special occasion' recipes that are more complicated. All oven temperatures are for preheated ovens, unless otherwise specified.

Recipes that have been included in the menu plans have been marked with an asterisk (*).

MICROWAVE COOKING

Just about all these dishes can be adapted to microwave cooking. Since my wife and I both have busy schedules, our microwave oven gets quite a workout; we cook practically every kind of food in it.

Microwaves vary somewhat, so check the instruction book that came with yours for specific directions on how to cook recipes similar to the ones in this book.

In general, roasts take about 13 minutes per pound (450 g), chops anything from 5 to 20 minutes depending on thickness and how many you are microwaving at once, while chicken pieces need about 3 minutes per piece. You can 'bake' a batch of muffins in a microwave in less than half the time a conventional oven takes, and the same is usually true of fish fillets. Our microwave oven cooks sliced vegetables in about 11 minutes per pound, and of course, you can have a tender baked potato on your plate in about 6 minutes using a microwave.

NUTRITIONAL ANALYSES

The nutritional contents of all the recipes were analysed using the ESHA Food Processor II computer programme. After each recipe, you will find information about calories, cholesterol, dietary fibre, fat and sodium content. Naturally, with the T-Factor Diet, you are primarily interested in watching your fat as well as your fibre intake, but the other amounts are provided for your information. If you are restricting your cholesterol and sodium intake, you will find these figures helpful.*

Cholesterol and sodium values were rounded up or down to the nearest whole milligram, while fat and fibre values were rounded up or down to the nearest half gram.

Herbs and spices have such minimal amounts of nutrients in the quantities used that they have been omitted from the analyses.

In recipes calling for beef, chicken or vegetable stock, the sodium content is estimated quite high because the computer program had only high-sodium bouillons in its database. I prefer homemade stock, and think it's well worth the minimal effort required to make it (see Basic Vegetable Stock, page 105, and Soup Base, page 106). Otherwise, I recommend looking for low-sodium or no-sodium consommés or stock cubes.

Since meat shrinks about 25 per cent in cooking we analysed the nutritional content of cooked meat. In recipes calling for chicken breasts, for example, we used a standard 3½ oz/100 g cooked chicken breast.

I hope you'll use these recipes not only for the sake of enjoying the tempting dishes themselves, but as guides to teach you how to modify your own favourite dishes to meet T-Factor standards.

* *Note for the British edition:* Because of differences in a small number of the ingredients available, these counts may vary slightly in a few recipes. Where this is at all significant, the discrepancy is pointed out.

BREAKFAST FOODS

Many nutritionists feel that breakfast is the most important meal of the day. After all, 'breakfast' means to 'break your fast'. When you wake in the morning you haven't eaten for many hours. If you're trying to lose weight, skipping breakfast can lead to bingeing later in the day because you may build up a 'hidden hunger'. As you will discover in Chapter Ten, it's the depletion of glycogen that stimulates your appetite. Breakfast can keep that depletion from prompting you to overeat. Here are some recipes that you can use to vary your standard breakfast routine.

These toppings can be used as spreads for toasted bread or muffins. They are especially good served on pancakes, for which one recipe follows.

Fruit Topping

8 fl oz/225 ml of fresh or unsweetened frozen berries or
other fruit
2 fl oz/55 ml of unsweetened
apple juice

1 teaspoon cornflour
Dash nutmeg, cinnamon
and/or ginger

1. Place the fruit in a saucepan. Stir the apple juice and cornflour together and pour over the fruit.
2. Heat over medium-low heat, stirring occasionally, until thickened. Add nutmeg or other spices to taste if desired. Serve hot.

Makes about 8 fl oz/225 ml: 4 servings of approx. 3 tablespoons
Per serving: 31 calories, 0 cholesterol, 1 g dietary fibre, 0 fat, 3 mg sodium

Strawberry-Banana Spread

8 oz/225 g strawberries
1 large ripe banana

Dash cinnamon or nutmeg

1. Mash together the berries and banana. Add the cinnamon and serve immediately, since bananas turn brown when they are left standing.

Makes about 8 fl oz/225 ml: 4 servings of approx. 3 tablespoons
Per serving: 38 calories, 0 cholesterol, 1.5 g dietary fibre, 0 fat, 1 mg sodium

Tropical Topping

8 fl oz/225 ml measure of sliced
  fresh or tinned apricots,
  unsweetened, drained
4 fl oz/110 ml crushed pineapple,
  unsweetened, drained

1 scant teaspoon of
  unsweetened grated coconut
1 teaspoon cornflour (optional)

1. Place the fruit in a blender or food processor and blend well. Pour the fruit into a saucepan, add the coconut, and heat through over medium-low heat, stirring occasionally.
2. Sprinkle with cornflour to thicken if desired, or serve as a syrup.

Makes about 12 fl oz/330 ml: 6 servings of about 3 tablespoons:
Per serving: 28 calories, 0 cholesterol, 1 g dietary fibre, 0 fat, 0 sodium

*Oatmeal Pancakes

5 oz/145 g oatmeal
16 fl oz/450 ml skimmed milk
1 egg
1 oz/28 g whole-wheat flour
3 tablespoons toasted
  wheatgerm

1 oz/28 g plain white flour
1 dessertspoon of baking
  powder
1½ teaspoons of sugar
1½ teaspoons of vegetable oil
½ teaspoon of salt

1. Combine the oats and milk and let stand for 10 minutes.
2. Stir in the remaining ingredients.
3. Heat a nonstick pan over medium-low heat. Pour 3 tablespoons of batter per pancake into the hot pan. Cook, turning once, until golden brown on both sides. Serve with one of the breakfast spreads immediately preceding.

Makes 12 pancakes
Per 2 pancakes: 179 calories, 47 mg cholesterol, 2 g dietary fibre, 4 g fat, 232 mg sodium

BREADS AND MUFFINS

Except for vitamin B_{12}, bread made from whole wheat has about the same vitamin and mineral content as beef (beef has more B_{12}). The average slice of whole-grain bread contains about 1 to 2 grams of fat, coming primarily from the grains themselves, not added fats. Also, the fibre content is much higher than in breads made with refined white flour. You will find, however, among the recipes that follow, some that call for a combination of white and whole-wheat flour, since whole-wheat flour alone tends to give a heavy consistency.

A slice of hot whole-grain bread or a muffin makes a great snack, so long as you don't smother it with butter or margarine! You will find your taste buds quickly adapting to unbuttered breads and muffins that are richly flavoured with whole grains and dried fruits.

Unless otherwise specified, all bread and muffin recipes call for preheated ovens.

Note for the British edition: American muffin-tins are about twice as deep as British tart- or bun-tins. They are available in this country and help you to produce a better product than the smaller British variety. If, however, you decide to use the smaller tins, each recipe quantity will make 24 small muffins and the portion size will become 2. The smaller tart- or bun-tins may be lined with paper cups. Because of their low fat content, muffins do not keep very well and you may wish, therefore, to halve the ingredients for some of the recipes or to freeze the baked muffins until required. They are worth trying – filling and very good.

Applesauce-Bran Muffins

You can vary this recipe by adding 2 oz/56 g sultanas or a diced apple after Step 4.

5 oz/145 g All Bran	1 oz/30 g butter or margarine,
8 fl oz/225 ml skimmed milk	melted
1 egg, slightly beaten	4 oz/110 g plain white flour
7 tablespoons unsweetened	2 teaspoons baking powder
apple sauce or stewed apple	2 level tablespoons brown sugar

1. Preheat oven to 400°F/Gas Mark 6/200°C. Lightly oil and flour muffin-tins.
2. In a large bowl, combine cereal and milk. Set aside.

3. In another bowl, combine egg, apple and melted butter. Stir into the cereal mixture.
4. Add the dry ingredients, stirring until just blended.
5. Fill each muffin-tin ¾ full.
6. Bake for 10–15 minutes or until nicely browned on top.

Makes 12 muffins.
Per muffin: 117 calories, 23 mg cholesterol, 4 g dietary fibre, 2.5 g fat, 238 mg sodium.

Gingersnap Muffins

5 oz/145 g whole-wheat flour	2 oz/56 g dates, chopped
1 dessertspoon baking powder	4 oz/110 g All Bran
½ teaspoon salt	12 fl oz/330 ml skimmed milk
2 dessertspoons brown sugar	3 level tablespoons molasses or
1 scant teaspoon ground ginger	black treacle
½ teaspoon cinnamon	1 large egg
¼ teaspoon ground cloves	2 desertspoons groundnut oil
2 oz/56 g raisins	

1. Preheat oven to 400°F/Gas Mark 6/200°C. Lightly oil and flour muffin-tins.
2. Measure bran cereal into a bowl or jug and combine with milk. Let stand.
3. Stir together flour, baking powder, salt, brown sugar, spices, raisins and dates in a large mixing bowl. Set aside.
4. In another jug, mix molasses, egg and peanut oil together until blended. Combine with cereal and milk mixture.
5. Pour the wet ingredients into the large mixing bowl with the dry ingredients and stir only until all is combined and moistened. Portion the batter evenly into tins.
6. Bake at 400 degrees for 18 to 20 minutes or until cooked through.

Makes 12 muffins.
Per muffin: 165 calories, 23 mg cholesterol, 5 g dietary fibre, 3 g fat, 297 mg sodium

Massachusetts Corn Muffins

7 tablespoons honey	2 oz/56 g sugar
2 whole eggs	2 dessertspoons baking powder
3 egg whites	14 oz/325 g plain white flour
14 fl oz/400 ml skimmed milk	5 oz/145 g maizemeal
3 tablespoons vegetable oil	¼ teaspoon salt

1. Preheat oven to 400°F/Gas Mark 6/200°C. Lightly oil and flour muffin-tins.
2. In a large bowl, whisk together the honey, eggs, egg whites, milk and oil.
3. Add the dry ingredients and mix with an electric mixer at medium-high speed for 2 minutes.
4. Fill baking cups ¾ full. Bake at 400 degrees for about 10–15 minutes, or until tops are golden brown.

Makes 24 muffins.
Per muffin: 155 calories, 23 mg cholesterol, 1 g dietary fibre, 3 g fat, 104 mg sodium.

Mixed Raisin-Bran Muffins

6 oz/175 g oat bran
4 oz/110 g whole-wheat cake and pastry flour
3 level tablespoons brown sugar
2 oz/156 g raisins
2 scant teaspoons baking powder
¼ teaspoon salt
8 fl oz/225 ml low-fat milk
1 egg, beaten
3 level tablespoons molasses or black treacle
2 dessertspoons vegetable oil

1. Preheat oven to 425°F/Gas Mark 7/220°C. Lightly oil and flour muffin-tins.
2. Combine dry ingredients in large bowl.
3. In separate bowl, mix milk, egg, molasses or black treacle and oil.
4. Add liquid ingredients to dry, and mix only until dry are moistened (the mixture should be lumpy).
5. Fill cups ¾ full, and bake at 425 degrees for 10–15 minutes, or until tops are golden brown.

Makes 12 muffins.
Per muffin: 192 calories, 25 mg cholesterol, 3 g dietary fibre, 3 g fat, 238 mg sodium.

No-Knead Peasant Bread

1 package (1 dessertspoon) traditional dry yeast
16 fl oz/450 ml lukewarm water
1 dessertspoon salt
1 dessertspoon sugar
12 oz/350 g whole-wheat bread flour
10–12 oz/285–350 g strong white flour
Maizemeal or whole-wheat flour
Water

1. Dissolve the yeast in the warm water. Add the salt and sugar and let stand for a minute or two.
2. Add the flours, 4 oz/110 g at a time, beating well after each addition, until dough becomes fairly stiff.
3. Shape dough into a ball and place in a bowl lightly greased with margarine or butter. Cover with plastic wrap and let rise in a warm place until doubled in bulk, about 1 hour.
4. Turn dough out on to a lightly floured board, knock down and shape into two long French-bread-style loaves, or into round loaves.
5. Place loaves on a baking sheet sprinkled heavily with maizemeal. Let rise 5 minutes.
6. Meanwhile, bring about 3 cups of water to a boil in an ovenproof pan.
7. Slash tops of loaves with a sharp knife. Brush loaves with cold water. Place them in a cold oven. Put the pan of boiling water in the oven on the rack below the bread. Turn oven to 400°F/Gas Mark 6/200°C and bake loaves about 45 minutes, until brown and crusty. Cool on a wire rack before slicing.

Makes 2 loaves, 10 slices each.
Per slice: 120 calories, 0 cholesterol, 2.5 g dietary fibre, 0.5 g fat, 321 mg sodium

Quick Whole-Wheat Buttermilk Bread

10 oz/300 g wholewheat bread flour
10 oz/300 g strong white flour
2 packages fast-action dry yeast
1½ oz/40 g wheatgerm
2 scant teaspoons baking powder

2 scant teaspoons salt
10 fl oz/275 mg buttermilk
6 fl oz/180 ml water
2 oz/56 g melted butter or margarine
2 dessertspoons molasses or black treacle

1. In a large bowl, mix together 6 oz/175 g of the whole-wheat flour, 6 oz/175 g white flour, the yeast, wheat germ, baking powder and salt.
2. In a saucepan, heat the buttermilk and water over medium-low heat until warm, not hot. Stir this into the flour mixture.
3. Melt the butter or margarine, and blend into the flour mixture. Blend in the molasses, and stir 100 strokes.
4. Slowly stir in the remaining whole-wheat flour and another 2 oz/56 g of the white flour. Add the remaining white flour in small amounts, mixing well after each addition.

5. Dust your kneading board, hands and dough with flour. Knead the dough for 8 to 10 minutes. Cover with a damp towel and set aside.
6. Grease two 2 lb/1 kg loaf-tins and preheat oven to 425°F/Gas Mark 7/220°C.
7. Divide the dough into 2 pieces. Pat each piece into a square of about 8 inches/20 cm, about 1 inch/2 cm thick. Fold the square in thirds. Seal the seam, and place each loaf, seam down, in a tin.
8. Cover with a damp towel and let rise until double in size, about 30 minutes.
9. Place the loaves in the centre of the oven and bake for 25 minutes, or until the loaves are nicely browned. Let cool on a wire rack.

Makes 2 loaves, 16 slices each.
Per slice: 86 calories, 4 mg cholesterol, 1 g dietary fibre, 2 g fat, 182 mg sodium.

Courgette Muffins

You can create an infinite number of variations on this recipe by substituting grated carrots for the courgettes, for example, or by using chopped fresh or dried fruit instead.

2 oz/56 g whole-wheat flour
2 oz/56 g plain white flour
2 scant teaspoons baking powder
½ teaspoon salt
4 oz/110 g sugar

1 egg white
4 fl oz/110 ml skimmed milk
1 dessertspoon melted butter or margarine
1 medium courgette, grated

1. Preheat oven to 375°F/Gas Mark 7/190°C. Lightly oil and flour muffin-tins.
2. Stir the dry ingredients together. Beat the egg white just until foamy. Add to the milk, along with the melted butter.
3. Add the liquid ingredients and the courgette to the dry ingredients, stirring just enough to moisten.
4. Pour into tins and bake for 10–20 minutes.

Makes 8 muffins.
Per muffin: 124 calories, 0 cholesterol, 1 g dietary fibre, 1.5 g fat, 247 mg sodium

LUNCHES

As a change from the basic lunches in the menu plans and as an alternative to high-fat, processed meats and cheeses, here are some sandwich spread ideas (you could also incorporate recipes from the Soups and Salads sections). And don't forget that cottage cheese is much more interesting for lunch when served with fresh fruit, salsa (Mexican-Style Hot Sauce, page 104), or jelly, or seasoned with Old Bay seasoning, Mrs. Dash, celery seed, garlic, or onion powder or a variety of other herbs and spices. For lunchtime salads, see page 146.

Crabmeat Spread

8 oz/225 g cooked crabmeat
2 stalks celery, diced small
1 small onion, diced small
Herb Salt to taste (page 153)
½ green pepper, diced

8 fl oz/225 ml measure bean sprouts
8 oz/225 g low-fat cottage cheese

Blend all the above ingredients with enough French dressing (oil and vinegar) to moisten.

Makes about 3 cups.
Per serving (3 tablespoons): 32 calories, 13 mg cholesterol, 0.5 g dietary fibre, 0.5 g fat, 215 mg sodium

Meat Spread

8 oz/225 g cooked meat or poultry
1 small onion, diced
3 tablespoons wheatgerm or cooked red beans

2 dessertspoons soya flour
Herb Salt (page 153) or other herb blend to taste
fresh-ground black pepper to taste

Blend all ingredients in a food processor. Moisten as needed with ketchup, mustard or French dressing.

Makes about 10 fl oz/275 ml.
Per serving (3 tablespoons): 99 calories, 38 mg cholesterol, 9.5 g dietary fibre, 2 g fat, 85 mg sodium

Mexican Bean Spread

This can also be used as a Mexican bean dip appetizer. It's great spread on a slice of whole-grain bread and grilled or baked in the oven with slices of tomato and some oregano.

15 oz/425 g tin dark-red kidney beans, drained
1 small onion
2 tablespoons tomato ketchup

⅛ teaspoon cayenne pepper
Herb Salt (page 153)
fresh-ground black pepper

Blend the above ingredients in a food processor, adding more ketchup if needed for desired consistency.

Makes about 12 fl oz/330 ml
Per serving (3 tablespoons): 78 calories, 0 cholesterol, 6 g dietary fibre, 0.5 g fat, 456 mg sodium

BEVERAGES

Research has shown that diet drinks are often the bane of over-weight people. Though low in calories and fat, drinking them tends to keep alive a taste for sweets, which can in turn lead to bingeing on fat-filled cakes and puddings. Studies have shown that people who drink diet drinks do *not* lose weight and keep it off as well as people who don't drink them.

My first recommendation for a no-cal beverage is WATER. Water is actually our most essential nutrient. We cannot live without it.

If, like many people, you can't stand the taste of tap water, it may be that the chemicals added in processing it in your town have ruined the taste. Either try bottled spring water or use a charcoal-activated, bacteriostatic filter to remove chlorine and other objectionable organic matter from your water.

I don't recommend drinking distilled water, as essential minerals have been removed.

Fruit and vegetable juices, herb teas and punches made from combinations of these are also good substitutes for soft drinks.

Coffee and black tea, of course, are standard no-cal beverages. Add a little milk if desired, and count up the fat grams accordingly. As long as you limit yourself to no more than two or three cups a day, you will probably suffer no ill effects from the caffeine. Because of increasing demand, many different coffees are now being decaffeinated, but if you use them, use water processed rather than those that are decaffeinated with methylene chloride. The package will carry the words 'water processed' if this process has been used. Methylene chloride is carcinogenic.

Iced Fruited Herb Tea

We like a combination of raspberry, apple, orange or lemon and mint teas in this drink.

8 herbal teabags – your choice	16 fl oz/450 ml orange juice
16 fl oz/450 ml boiling water	1¾ pints/1 litre cold water

1. Soak the tea bags in the boiling water for 20 to 30 minutes.
2. In a large jug, combine the orange juice and cold water. Remove the teabags and add the hot tea to the juice mixture. Stir. Chill for at least 1 hour.

Makes 8 servings.
Per serving: 56 calories, 0 cholesterol, 0.5 g dietary fibre, 0 fat, 1 mg sodium

Spiced Tea

Pre-mixed instant teas and lemonades are usually high in sugar as well as other additives. Here is a tangy alternative that lets you control the amount of sugar. Serve hot or cold.

1¾ pints/1 litre brewed
  black tea
2 cinnamon sticks
8 fl oz/225 ml unsweetened
  orange juice

1–1½ teaspoons sugar
1 scant teaspoon ground
  cloves
1–2 teaspoons lemon juice,
  or 4 slices fresh lemon

1. When brewing the tea, place the cinnamon sticks in the same pan or teapot. When the tea is ready, discard the cinnamon sticks.
2. Add the remaining ingredients to the pot and serve, or chill first in a pitcher and serve over ice cubes if you want iced tea.

Makes 4 servings.
Per serving: 38 calories, 0 cholesterol, 0 dietary fibre, 0 fat, 9 mg sodium

APPETIZERS AND SNACKS

One of my favourite appetizers when we have guests is simply a variety of fresh fruits. However, here are a few recipes for dips, chips and more that are suitable for both snacks and parties. On occasions when you are going to be a guest at someone's house, you might ask if you may bring an appetizer. Then you can be sure that there'll be at least one low-fat food available.

Chickpea Dip

1 lb 4 oz/600 g cooked chickpeas, drained
3 dessertspoons tahini (sesame seed paste)
2 fl oz/50ml lemon juice

3 cloves garlic, crushed
1 spring onion or shallot, minced
dash salt
parsley sprigs

1. Combine all ingredients except parsley in a blender or food processor and blend into a thick paste. Pour into serving bowl and chill.
2. Garnish with parsley and serve with whole-grain crispbreads or raw fresh vegetables.

Makes about 40 dessertspoons.
Per 2 dessertspoons: 62 calories, 0 cholesterol, 2 g dietary fibre, 2 g fat, 13 mg sodium

Herb Dip

Serve this with toasted pita bread triangles, whole-grain crispbreads, or cut up fresh vegetables. Or try it on a baked potato instead of sour cream.

8 fl oz/225 ml plain low-fat yoghurt
¼ teaspoon garlic powder
⅛ teaspoon dill weed
¼ teaspoon oregano

¼ teaspoon basil
½ teaspoon chives
½ teaspoon dried parsley
½ teaspoon marjoram
dash of salt

Combine all ingredients in a medium-sized mixing bowl. Chill for a couple of hours before serving.

Makes 8 fl oz/225 ml.
Per 2 fl oz/50 ml: 32 calories, 1 mg cholesterol, 0 dietary fibre, 0 fat, 123 mg sodium

Home-Made Tortilla Chips

Keep your eye on these while they are baking, as they brown quickly.

1 or 2 dessertspoons vegetable oil	1 package corn tortillas (10 tortillas)*

1. Spread part of the oil lightly on a foil-covered baking sheet with a pastry brush.
2. Stack the tortillas on top of one another and cut into eighths. Spread the tortilla pieces on the baking sheet, and brush lightly with oil.
3. Bake at 350°F/Gas Mark 5/180°C for about 10 minutes, or until just beginning to turn crispy and brown.

Variations: Sprinkle the chips with garlic powder, Parmesan cheese, paprika or other seasonings before baking.

Makes 80 chips.

Per chip (made with tortillas): 10 calories, 0 cholesterol, 0 dietary fibre, 0.5 g fat, 2 mg sodium

* If tortillas are not readily available, try Indian pappadoms cut with scissors and placed for a minute or two under a hot grill.

*Mexican-Style Hot Sauce (Salsa)

This is a good dip for Home-Made Tortilla Chips (above), or any Mexican recipe. It also adds spice to cottage cheese. It requires no cooking and contains no oil. We like it spicy-hot, but if you prefer a milder sauce, cut back on the Tabasco ... or the crushed red pepper ... or the jalapeños!

28 oz/800 g tin whole tomatoes	2 tablespoons juice from jalapeños
5–6 oz/145–75 g tin tomato paste	
4 spring onions, finely chopped	1 dessertspoon Tabasco sauce
½ medium sweet pepper, diced	1 dessertspoon crushed red pepper
1–4 jalapeño peppers, finely chopped	
	6 fl oz/180 ml water

1. Pour the whole tomatoes into a large bowl, along with their juice. Chop the tomatoes into small pieces.
2. Add all the other ingredients, blending well. Store in a glass container in the refrigerator (you must use glass because the acid in the peppers will react with metal or plastic).

Makes about 2½ pints/1.3 litres.

Per dessertspoon: 4 calories, 0 cholesterol, 0 dietary fibre, 0 fat, 2 mg sodium

SOUPS

Some studies have shown that people who often include soup with their meals find it easier to lose weight and maintain their losses. Clear soups are generally lower in fat than cream soups, but you can make low-fat 'cream' soups by substituting skimmed milk for the cream or whole milk, with perhaps some skimmed dried milk, flour or cornflour added to make the soup richer and thicker.

I include some recipes for stock, as I like to use my own in recipes calling for bouillon or consommé. You can also save any water used for steaming vegetables to use as vegetable stock in other recipes. I use commercial brands at a pinch, but they tend to be much higher in sodium and preservatives. So, in my family, we make a potful of stock and freeze part of it for later use. Try adapting your own favourite soup recipes by cutting fat and experimenting with seasonings.

Basic Vegetable Stock

Here's a basic recipe for a stock made from water and a variety of fresh vegetables. You can add other vegetables, such as parsnips, turnips, leeks, etc., if desired.

3 medium carrots, cut in chunks	1 bay leaf
2 stalks celery, cut in chunks	6 whole peppercorns
3 medium onions, cut in chunks	½ teaspoon tarragon and/or other dried herbs
3 cloves garlic, minced	2½ pints/1.3 litres water
small handful fresh parsley, chopped	

1. Combine all ingredients in a large saucepan, and bring to a boil. Reduce heat to simmer, cover, and let cook for about 1 hour.
2. You may strain the vegetables out and use the clear bouillon, or put the stock in a blender and puree for a thicker stock, adding a bit more water if necessary.

Makes about 3 pints/2 litres.
Per 8 fl oz/225 ml: 24 calories, 0 cholesterol, 2 g dietary fibre, 0 fat, 23 mg sodium

Soup Base

This basic stock can be used for making all kinds of soups, and for cooking rice and other grains and boiled potatoes. It is excellent for soaking and cooking beans.

Save all chicken and turkey giblets (necks, hearts, gizzards, but *not* livers). Freeze these parts immediately, first trimming skin and any fat from the necks, and hold in your freezer until you have the giblets of 4–6 birds.

You may substitute a beef soup bone or two for the giblets, but I prefer the lighter flavour and lower cholesterol of chicken stock.

giblets of 4–6 birds
1 large bay leaf
salt and pepper to taste
1 teaspoon each: rosemary, sage, thyme, tarragon
1 large onion, coarsely chopped

2 large stalks celery, cut in 2 inch/5 cm pieces (include leaves)
2 large carrots, cut in 2 inch/5 cm pieces

1. Place the giblets in a deep saucepan, with enough water to cover (about 3–4 pints/2–2.5 litres). Bring to a boil and skim as necessary. When finally clear of scum, add the remaining ingredients. You may also throw in any other greens or wilted vegetables you have on hand in your refrigerator (except for asparagus, cabbage, broccoli or cauliflower, which taste too strong).
2. Bring to a boil once again, then reduce heat and simmer for at least 2 hours.
3. Separate the giblets and vegetables from the water. Blend the vegetables in a blender or food processor until smooth, and return to the stock. Save the cooked giblets for low-calorie snacks.

Makes about 4 pints/2½ litres, depending on how many giblets and vegetables you add. If there is too much for your needs over the next few days (stored in the refrigerator), freeze some in plastic tubs.
Per 8 fl oz/225 ml approx: 31 calories, 20 mg cholesterol, 1 g dietary fibre, 0.5 g fat, 82 mg sodium

*Broccoli Soup

This wholesome, nutrient-rich soup warms any evening. Use as a main course topped with 2 dessertspoons of grated cheese and croutons. As a starter or a snack, skip the cheese. You can also make Cauliflower Soup by substituting 2 pounds/900 g of cauliflower for the broccoli. Add a dessertspoon of lemon juice for tanginess.

1½ lb/675 g broccoli, stalks separated
16 fl oz/450 ml water
2 stalks celery, chopped
1 onion, chopped
1 dessertspoon olive oil
2 dessertspoons flour

1 pint/570 ml water
1 chicken stock cube
⅛ teaspoon pepper
⅛ teaspoon nutmeg
4 fl oz/110 ml evaporated skimmed milk

1. Heat the 16 fl oz/450 ml of water in a large pan till boiling.
2. Add vegetables, cover and cook till tender (about 10 minutes).
3. Blend vegetables with part of the cooking water in a blender or food processor.
4. Heat olive oil in a small non-stick pan. Add 2 tablespoons of the 2½ cups of water and sprinkle in the flour. Cook and stir until smooth.
5. Add the remaining water and heat to boiling, stirring constantly. Boil and stir 1 minute.
6. Stir in broccoli mixture, stock cube, pepper, and nutmeg. Heat just until boiling.
7. Stir in the evaporated skimmed milk and heat through without boiling again.

Makes about 9 servings.
Per serving: 86 calories, 1 mg cholesterol, 5 g dietary fibre, 3 g fat, 371 mg sodium

*Corn Chowder

6 spring onions, chopped
1 teaspoon oil
1 pint/570 ml chicken stock
16 fl oz/450 ml skimmed milk
1¼ lb/575 g potatoes, cubed
2 packages (10 oz/300 g each) frozen sweetcorn

3 tablespoons skimmed instant dried milk
¼ teaspoon dry mustard
⅛ teaspoon salt
pinch to ⅛ teaspoon black pepper

1. Sauté onions in oil in a large non-stick saucepan. Add chicken stock, milk and potatoes. Bring to a boil, lower heat and simmer until potatoes are tender, about 12 minutes. Add sweetcorn and cook 1 minute more.
2. Remove about a third of the chowder to a food processor. Purée and return to saucepan.
3. Stir in dried milk, mustard, salt and pepper. Serve immediately.

Makes 8 cups
Per cup: 165 calories, 3 mg cholesterol, 4 g dietary fibre, 2 g fat, 397 mg sodium

*Gazpacho

Serve this soup chilled in bowls with one of the following assortment of garnishes: chopped hard-boiled egg, finely chopped spring onions, chives or croutons.

1 large tomato	2 tablespoons red wine vinegar
½ small onion	4 fl oz/110 ml white wine
½ cucumber	2 dessertspoons basil
½ green pepper	1 dessertspoon lemon juice
1 celery stalk	1 scant teaspoon salt
2 teaspoons fresh parsley, finely chopped	½ teaspoon white pepper
2 cloves garlic, minced or crushed	1 scant teaspoon Worcestershire sauce
16 fl oz/450 ml tomato juice	dash of Tabasco sauce

Finely chop all vegetables. (A food processor is ideal for this.) Combine with all remaining ingredients and refrigerate 24 hours.

Makes about 4½ servings.
Per serving: 42 calories, 0 cholesterol, 2 g dietary fibre, 0 fat, 658 mg sodium (analyses are without garnishes)

*Minestrone

1 medium onion, chopped	4 oz/110 g uncooked macaroni (try whole-wheat)
1 stalk celery, chopped	
2 medium carrots, chopped	15 oz/425 g tin navy beans with juice
8 oz/225 g fresh or frozen french beans	
	¼ teaspoon basil
1 medium courgette, chopped	¼ teaspoon oregano
10 oz/300 g package frozen chopped spinach	¼ teaspoon cayenne pepper
	water as needed.
28 oz/800 g tin tomatoes	

Combine all ingredients in a large pot. Bring to a boil, then reduce heat and let simmer for about 30 minutes, until all vegetables are tender. Add water if necessary to make enough liquid to cover ingredients.

Makes about 12 cups.
Per 1½ cups: 137 calories, 0 cholesterol, 7.5 g dietary fibre, 1 g fat, 207 mg sodium

Potato-Vegetable Soup

This is a fast soup – that is, it takes 10 minutes to get everything into the pot. It is a prototype for any quick soup. Just start with stock and add any vegetables, potatoes, rice, lentils or other grains or legumes, and cook for 1 hour.

16 fl oz/450 ml stock
1 medium potato, cut in eighths
1 onion, sliced
3 carrots, sliced

2 stalks celery, sliced
½ teaspoon fresh-ground black pepper
1 dessertspoon dried parsley

Place all ingredients in a large saucepan. Bring to a boil, reduce heat, and cook over low heat for 1 hour.

Makes 4 servings.
Per serving (8 fl oz/225 ml): 91 calories, 0 cholesterol, 3 g dietary fibre, 0.5 g fat, 387 mg sodium

**Split-Pea Soup*

A warming crowd-pleaser. Halve the recipe for a smaller crowd! If you like a smooth-textured soup, you may whir it in a blender or pass it through a sieve.

2 lb/900 g dried split peas
7 pints/4 litres meat or vegetable stock
3 carrots, sliced thin
2 onions, chopped
6 stalks celery, chopped

½ teaspoon black pepper
1 scant teaspoon salt
½ teaspoon thyme
2 cloves garlic, minced
⅛ teaspoon cayenne
2 dessertspoons flour (optional)

1. Cook peas in stock for 2½ hours.
2. Add remaining ingredients and cook for 1 additional hour. You may thicken the soup by sprinkling in the flour and blending well.

Serves 16.
Per serving (8 fl oz/225 ml): 178 calories, 0 cholesterol, 8 g dietary fibre, 0.5 g fat, 393 mg sodium

FISH

The many different varieties of fish are usually quick and easy to prepare in a number of delicious, low-fat ways: poaching, steaming, baking and grilling. Watch cooking times carefully to avoid overcooking.

As an added bonus, fish also contains 'Omega III' fatty acids that can reduce the risk of heart disease. One of these, eicosapentanoic acid (EPA), has been shown to lower serum cholesterol and triglycerides and to increase high-density lipoproteins (HDL). Lower total cholesterol and higher HDL levels are both associated with a reduced risk of cardiovascular disease. EPA also lessens the risk of blood clots and strokes by causing some changes in the red blood cells and platelets in the bloodstream that are responsible for clotting.

The best sources of Omega III fatty acids are cold-water fish: salmon, mackerel, bluefish, albacore tuna and herring. Moderate amounts can be found in halibut, red snapper, swordfish and shellfish, while cod and monkfish have a little less. Although the fish richest in Omega III fatty acids contain more fat than other varieties, they are still generally lower in fat than red meat. Flounder, plaice, haddock and sole, for example, may be very low in fat, but the health benefits and reasonable fat contents of the fattier fish listed above recommend their use on a regular basis.

*Grilled Tuna Mediterranean

Marinade:

1 dessertspoon capers	½ teaspoon dried rosemary, crushed
1 dessertspoon olive oil	
3 dessertspoons white wine	¼ teaspoon salt
2 dessertspoons lemon juice	fresh-ground black pepper to taste
1 clove garlic, crushed	

1 lb/450 g fresh tuna steaks, about ½ to ¾ inch/1 to 2 cm thick	1 teaspoon of olive oil
	Lemon wedges
	Fresh parsley sprigs

1. Place capers in a strainer and rinse under cold running water. Drain well.
2. Combine all marinade ingredients in shallow glass or ceramic dish. Arrange the tuna steaks in the dish and marinate for 20 minutes, turning once after 10 minutes.

3. Brush a foil-lined grill pan with oil and arrange the marinated tuna steaks on the sheet. Pour half the marinade over the steaks.
4. Grill the fish for about 4 minutes, until the tops are slightly seared. Turn the steaks over with a spatula and pour the remaining marinade over them. Grill another 4 minutes, or until fish flakes easily with a fork.
5. Garnish each serving with lemon wedges and fresh parsley.

Makes 4 servings.
Per serving: 173 calories, 53 mg cholesterol, 0 dietary fibre, 9 g fat, 134 mg sodium

Lime-steamed Fish Fillets

These basic directions can be used whenever you want to steam fish.

1½ lb/675 g fish fillets (try flounder or sole)
juice of 1 lime

2 shallots, minced
fresh-ground black pepper to taste

1. Arrange fillets on a steamer rack over boiling water.
2. Squeeze the lime juice over them, and top with shallots and black pepper.
3. Cover and steam for about 5 minutes, until fish flakes easily with a fork.

Makes 4 servings.
Per serving: 124 calories, 66 mg cholesterol, 0.5 g dietary fibre, 2 g fat, 155 mg sodium

Royal Indian Salmon

This recipe is one of our all-time favourites, delicately flavoured and very easy to prepare.

4 salmon steaks, 1 inch/2.5 cm thick
3 tablespoons low-sodium chicken or vegetable bouillon
2 dessertspoons lemon juice
½ teaspoon fennel seeds, crushed

¼ teaspoon cumin
¼ teaspoon ground coriander
dash of salt and fresh-ground black pepper

1. Place the salmon steaks in a shallow glass or china dish. Pour the bouillon and the lemon juice over and add the seasonings. Marinate, covered, in the refrigerator for at least 2 hours, turning the steaks occasionally.
2. To cook, place the steaks on a foil-covered grill pan. Spoon 2 teaspoons of the marinade on top of each steak. Place under the grill at low heat for 8 to 10 minutes, or until slightly brown on the edges. Turn steaks over, spoon on the remaining marinade, and grill for an additional 8 to 10 minutes.

Makes 4 servings, about 4½ oz/125 g each, cooked weight
Per serving: 285 calories, 120 mg cholesterol, 0 dietary fibre, 8 g fat, 225 mg sodium

Salmon Croquettes Béarnaise

A traditional favourite. Serve with Light Béarnaise Sauce (page 151).

15 oz/425 g tin salmon	1 dessertspoon lemon juice
½ onion, finely chopped	¼ teaspoon pepper
9 tablespoons breadcrumbs	¼ teaspoon nutmeg
1 egg, slightly beaten	

1. Combine all ingredients in a bowl and mix well.
2. Cover and refrigerate the salmon mixture for an hour or more.
3. After chilling, shape into 4 patties approximately ¾ inch/2 cm thick.
4. Lightly oil a non-stick frying pan and fry the patties over moderate heat, turning once, until browned on each side.

Makes 4 servings.
Per serving: 173 calories, 90 mg cholesterol, 1 g dietary fibre, 5.5 g fat, 433 mg sodium

Saucy Seafood Kebabs

This recipe is delicious with halibut, which holds together well during cooking, but other fish steaks or fillets can be used.

1 lb/450 g fish, cut into 1 inch/2 cm cubes	8 fl oz/225 ml tomato juice
16 cherry tomatoes	1 tablespoon cider vinegar
2 sweet peppers, cut into 1 inch/2 cm cubes	½ teaspoon dry mustard
16 mushrooms	¼ teaspoon garlic powder
16 cooked white pearl onions	large pinch black pepper
	small pinch cayenne pepper

1. Thread the raw fish alternately with the vegetables on four skewers. Place the kebabs on a lightly oiled grill pan.
2. Place the remaining ingredients in a saucepan and heat through.
3. Brush the heated sauce on the kebabs. Grill the kebabs about 3 inches/7 cm away from the heat for 12 to 15 minutes, turning once halfway through the cooking time. Baste the kebabs with the remaining sauce occasionally while cooking.

Makes 4 servings.
Per serving (using lemon sole): 160 calories, 68 mg cholestrol, 5 g dietary fibre, 2 g fat 322 mg sodium

Sea Bass with Red Peppers

This is also good made with haddock or other thick fillets of fish.

1 lb/450 g bass fillets
1 tablespoon fresh parsley, minced
¼ teaspoon chives
¼ teaspoon marjoram
¼ teaspoon tarragon
⅛ teaspoon rosemary

juice of ¼ lemon
4 fl oz/110 ml white wine
4 large mushrooms, sliced thinly
1 small red sweet pepper, diced
2 tablespoons dry breadcrumbs
1 teaspoon butter

1. Place fish fillets in a shallow baking dish. Sprinkle with the seasonings and lemon juice. Pour the wine around the fish. Arrange the vegetables in the liquid around the fish.
2. Bake at 400°/Gas Mark 6/200°C for 15 minutes.
3. Stir the vegetables. Sprinkle the breadcrumbs on the fish and dot with the butter. Cook 15 minutes more.

Makes 4 servings.
Per serving: 148 calories, 83 mg cholesterol, 1 g dietary fibre, 2.5 g fat, 160 mg sodium

Shrimps Florentine

1 onion, chopped
1 dessertspoon butter
2 tablespoons water
2 large cloves garlic, minced
1 sweet pepper, chopped
16 fl oz/450 ml stock (chicken or fish)
8 oz/225 g uncooked brown rice

fresh-ground black pepper to taste
10 oz/300 g package frozen chopped spinach
1 teaspoon soy sauce
1 lb/450 g shrimps, cooked and peeled
salt to taste

1. Cook onion in butter and water in a saucepan over low heat until onion is translucent. Add the garlic and cook until lightly browned. Add the pepper, cover, and gently steam until somewhat tender. Remove from heat.
2. Meanwhile, bring the stock to a boil in another saucepan. Rinse the rice and add it to the boiling stock. Cover, reduce heat to simmer, and let cook about 40 minutes or until rice is tender. Sprinkle with black pepper.
3. In another pan, cook the spinach in water, as directed on the package. Add the lemon juice and soy sauce.
4. Add the shrimps to the onion and pepper mixture and toss. Heat gently until heated through.
5. To serve, spoon rice onto a plate, top with spinach and then the shrimp mixture. Season with extra soy sauce or salt as desired.

Makes 4 servings.
Per serving: 368 calories, 175 mg cholesterol, 4.5 g dietary fibre, 6.5 g fat, 768 mg sodium

Simple Fish in Foil

A delicious and simple use for those fish fillets in the freezer!

1 lb/450 g frozen fish fillets
¼ teaspoon dried dill weed
1½ tablespoons lemon juice
4 slices onion
2 medium potatoes, cut into
  ¼ inch/½ cm strips

2 medium carrots, cut into
  thin slices
8 oz/225 g frozen Italian
  green beans

1. Place each frozen fish fillet in the centre of an individual piece of foil, 12 × 18 inches/30 × 45 cm.
2. Combine dill and lemon juice. Drizzle over fillets.
3. Top with onion slices. Arrange potatoes and carrots beside the fillets. Top with green beans.
4. Seal foil tightly and place on ungreased baking sheet.
5. Bake at 450°F/Gas Mark 7/220°C till fork tender, about 30 minutes.

Makes 4 servings.
Per serving: 189 calories, 59 mg cholesterol, 3 g dietary fibre, 1.5 g fat, 157 mg sodium

*Oysters Rockefeller

2 tablespoons of dry
 breadcrumbs
1½ teaspoons of olive oil
1 dessertspoon of grated onion
Tarragon, pepper, and/or
 Tabasco sauce to taste
1 package (10 oz/280 g) of
chopped frozen spinach,
 thawed and drained
6 oz/170 g of raw or tinned
 oysters (not smoked)
2 dessertspoons grated low-fat
 mozzarella cheese
1 dessertspoon of Parmesan

1. Combine the breadcrumbs, oil, onion, and seasonings. Toss
   together with the spinach.
2. Grill the oysters, if using raw, for 5 to 7 minutes. Drain liquid if
   using tinned.
3. Top oysters with spinach mixture and grill 3 to 4 minutes.
   Sprinkle with the cheeses and grill until just melted.

Makes 4 servings.
Per serving: 103 calories, 24 mg cholesterol, 2.5 g dietary fibre, 4.5 g
fat, 169 mg sodium

Swordfish with Tarragon

4 swordfish steaks, 6–8 oz/
 175–225 g each
1 dessertspoon olive oil
1 dessertspoon lemon juice
1½ teaspoons tarragon
2 dessertspoons grated Parmesan cheese
1 teaspoon paprika

1. In a foil-covered baking dish, swish the fish in the olive oil and
   lemon juice to coat both sides. Grill 4 to 5 minutes on each side.
2. Meanwhile, combine the remaining ingredients in a small bowl.
   Sprinkle the fish with the seasoning mixture in the last minute of
   cooking time.

Makes 4 servings.
Per serving: 228 calories, 68 mg cholesterol, 0 dietary fibre, 8.5 g fat,
158 mg sodium

BEEF

Although beef is high in saturated fat as compared to poultry and seafood, I eat low-fat cuts in moderation (once or twice a week). I don't feel there is strong evidence against eating it even three to four times a week, provided your cholesterol level is normal and there is no history of heart disease in your family.

The low-fat cuts of beef are topside and silverside, sirloin tip, flank steak, fillet and, of course, extra-lean mince. However, all prepared mince contains a percentage of fat. For truly lean mince, ask your butcher to mince a lean cut for you while you wait.

Trim all visible fat from other cuts of beef before cooking, and try using beef as a condiment combined with lots of vegetables, as in Oriental cooking.

*Baked Flank Steak

1½ lb/675 g flank steak
1 dessertspoon vegetable oil
8 fl oz/225 ml hot water
1 bay leaf
1 large clove garlic, crushed
1 scant teaspoon salt

3 tablespoons minced celery
⅛ teaspoon black pepper
2 teaspoons lemon juice
1 medium carrot, diced
¼ medium sweet pepper, diced

1. Trim away any visible fat from the steak. Sear the steak in the oil over medium to medium-high heat. Place the steak in a casserole dish.
2. For extra flavouring, pour the water into the pan in which you seared the meat, and stir. Pour this over the meat, then add all the other ingredients.
3. Cook uncovered at 350°F/Gas Mark 5/180°C for 30 minutes, or longer if you prefer your meat well done.

Light Gravy (Optional): Heat 1 dessertspoon of vegetable oil and stir in 2 dessertspoons of whole-wheat flour. Slowly add the liquid from the meat as you stir. Stir until thickened, and serve over the meat.

Makes 4 servings, 4½ oz/125 g each, plus sauce, but without optional gravy. Per serving: 273 calories, 88 mg cholesterol, 1 g dietary fibre, 12 g fat, 630 mg sodium (gravy adds 30 calories and 3 grams of fat; nutrient values of the meat liquid and other ingredients are included in the original analysis)

Chilli-Bean Meat Loaf

2 lb/900 g cooked red kidney
  beans
1 lb/450 g lean mince
2 oz/56 g dry breadcrumbs
2 dessertspoons soy sauce

½ teaspoon dried oregano
1 dessertspoon dried basil
15 oz/430 g tin tomato purée or
  chopped tomatoes
dash cayenne pepper

1. Preheat oven to 350°F/Gas Mark 5/180°C.
2. Drain the liquid from the kidney beans.
3. Mix half the beans with the meat, breadcrumbs, soy sauce, oregano and basil.
3. Press mixture into a 9 × 5 × 3 inch/23 × 12 × 7 cm loaf-tin, and cover with the remaining beans and the tomato purée. Sprinkle with cayenne pepper.
4. Bake uncovered for 1 hour.

Makes 8 servings.
Per serving: 252 calories, 38 mg cholesterol, 8 g dietary fibre, 9 g fat, 761 mg sodium

Chinese Beef with Vegetables

1 teaspoon groundnut oil
2 teaspoons water
12 oz/350 g topside, trimmed of
  fat, cut diagonally into thin
  strips
1 medium onion, chopped
¼ teaspoon ground ginger
2 heads broccoli, chopped

2 carrots, sliced
8 fl oz/225 ml beef stock
4 oz/110 g mange tout peas
4 oz/110 g water chestnuts,
  drained and sliced
4 oz/110 g bean sprouts
1 dessertspoon soy sauce
1 dessertspoon cornflour

1. Place oil and water in large lidded frying pan or wok and heat over medium-high heat. Add meat and onion and brown lightly. Add remaining ingredients except soy sauce and cornflour. Cover and cook until vegetables are just tender.
2. Mix the soy sauce and cornflour together to make a paste. Stir into the other ingredients and cook, stirring occasionally, until thickened. Serve with brown rice.

Makes 4 servings.
Per serving: 201 calories, 61 mg cholesterol, 4.5 g dietary fibre, 8 g fat, 160 mg sodium (analyses do not include the rice, which is generally 1 gram of fat per 3 heaped tablespoons).

Japanese Beef Stir-Fry

Serve this dish as soon as it's ready, or, if you are making enough for leftovers, use white or Chinese cabbage instead of red, as the red cabbage tends to turn other ingredients purple when cooked and stored.

4 beef fillet steaks (about 4 oz/110 g each)
1 dessertspoon groundnut oil
12 oz/350 g mange tout peas
¼ head red cabbage, sliced thinly

¼ inch/½ cm fresh ginger root, minced, or ground ginger to taste
1 dessertspoon sake (optional)
dash tamari or low-sodium soy sauce

1. Heat a wok or heavy frying pan over medium-high heat for several minutes. Meanwhile, trim the beef of all visible fat and slice it into thin slices.
2. Add the oil to the pan, then the beef. Cook, stirring constantly, until browned.
3. Turn the heat down to medium, remove the meat from the pan, and set aside.
4. Add the cabbage, ginger root and mange tout to the wok, and cook for 5 minutes, stirring constantly.
5. Return the meat to the wok, and stir in the sake and the soy sauce. Cover, and let simmer for a few more minutes, until the vegetables are just tender and the meat is cooked the way you like it.

Makes 4 servings.
Per serving: 281 calories, 82 mg cholesterol, 8 g dietary fibre, 13 g fat, 81 mg sodium

Pot Roast

2 lb/900 g lean beef cut into 2 inch/5 cm cubes
3 onions, sliced
4 cloves garlic, chopped
1 sweet pepper, sliced
4 large stalks celery, cut into 2 inch/5 cm pieces
6 medium carrots, cut into 2 inch/5 cm pieces
2 lb/900 g potatoes, cut into eighths

1 large tin (1 lb 12 oz/800 g) whole tomatoes
1 tin (15 oz/425 g) tomato sauce or tomato purée
1 dessertspoon soy sauce
1 teaspoon Worcestershire sauce
8 fl oz/225 ml stock
1 dessertspoon dried basil
fresh-ground black pepper to taste

1. Place meat, onions, garlic, pepper, celery, carrots and potatoes in large roasting pan.
2. Cover with tinned tomatoes, tomato sauce, soy sauce, Worcestershire sauce and stock. Sprinkle with basil and ground black pepper.
3. Cook in a covered pan at 350°F/Gas Mark 5/180°C for 45 minutes. Reduce heat to 250°F/Gas Mark ½/130°C and cook for 3 hours or until meat is very tender to the fork. Baste occasionally.

Makes 6 servings of 4 oz/110 g of beef (cooked weight) each with assorted vegetables.
Per serving: 473 calories, 78 mg cholesterol, 8 g dietary fibre, 8 g fat, 667 mg sodium

Round Roast Oriental

3 lb/1.3 kg topside or silverside	1 tablespoon mustard powder
1 large clove garlic, crushed	1 dessertspoon tamari or low-sodium soy sauce
2 more large cloves garlic, cut in half	2 teaspoons toasted sesame seeds, crushed
2 dessertspoons sake or sherry	8 fl oz/225 ml water or stock
1 dessertspoon honey	

1. Trim all visible fat from the beef, then rub the beef all over with the crushed garlic. Cut four slits in the roast and insert a piece of peeled, sliced garlic clove into each slit. Place in a roasting pan.
2. Combine the remaining ingredients in a small bowl and pour over the roast. Let marinate at room temperature for 1 hour.
3. Bake, covered, at 350°F/Gas Mark 5/180°C for 2 hours, or until done, basting occasionally. Remove the garlic cloves before serving, unless you like a lot of garlic!

Makes 12 servings, 3 oz each
Per serving: 207 calories, 82 mg cholesterol, 0 dietary fibre, 9 g fat, 136 mg sodium

*Saucy Pastitiso

8 oz/225 g very lean mince
1 onion, chopped
8 fl oz/225 ml tomato sauce
¼ teaspoon salt
¼ teaspoon pepper
⅛ teaspoon cinnamon
⅛ teaspoon allspice
⅛ teaspoon nutmeg

8 oz/225 g elbow pasta or
   macaroni, cooked according
   to package directions
2 dessertspoons grated Parmesan cheese
10 fl oz/275 ml skimmed or
   semi-skimmed milk
2 dessertspoons flour
3 drops Tabasco

1. Lightly oil an 8 × 8 × 1½ inch/20 × 20 × 1 cm baking tin. Preheat oven to 375°F/Gas Mark 5/190°C.
2. Oil a medium-sized non-stick frying pan. Brown meat and onion in hot pan for 3 minutes or until meat is no longer pink. Pour off and discard any excess fat. Stir in tomato sauce, ⅛ teaspoon of the salt, ⅛ teaspoon of the pepper, the cinnamon, allspice and nutmeg into meat mixture. Stir in hot cooked elbow macaroni and Parmesan cheese. Spoon into prepared baking pan.
3. Stir together milk and flour in a medium saucepan until very smooth. Bring to a boil. Lower heat and cook 1 minute or until mixture thickens slightly. Stir in Tabasco and the remaining salt and pepper. Pour white sauce over meat mixture in baking pan.
4. Bake for 25 minutes or until centre is hot. Serve with a crisp mixed green salad, if you wish.

Makes 4 servings.
Per serving: 395 calories, 39 mg cholesterol, 3 g dietary fibre, 10 g fat, 259 mg sodium

Steak Marinades

Here are two marinades for flank steak or any other lean cut of beef that you might want to use for roasting, grilling or a barbecue. The wine and soy sauce have a tenderizing effect, so marinate overnight in the refrigerator, in a large covered bowl or plastic bag. Turn the meat once or twice while it is marinating, to be sure all of it has been well covered.

These amounts will do nicely for 2 pounds/900 g of meat.

Basic marinade:

1 dessertspoon olive oil
4 fl oz/110 ml dry red wine
  (you can use white wine for
  light-coloured meats)
¼ teaspoon Herb Salt (page
  153)
1 bay leaf
1 teaspoon chives
1 small onion, minced

Oriental marinade:

1 dessertspoon olive oil
3 tablespoons tamari (or soy
  sauce)
3 tablespoons dry red wine
4 cloves garlic, minced
4 spring onions, minced
6 whole peppercorns
⅛ teaspoon ground coriander
1 inch/2 cm cube fresh ginger,
  peeled and grated or minced

Olive oil contains approximately 120 calories and 12 grams of fat per dessertspoon. The other ingredients provide negligible calories, including the wine, since the alcohol will evaporate and the sugar content is very low. Soy sauce is quite high in sodium, but it is difficult to predict how much will penetrate or adhere to the meat. My guess is that the sodium content per serving, for example, 4½ oz/125 g of flank steak, would be moderate, perhaps 500 milligrams.

Swedish Meatballs

Here is an example of how you can adapt your favourite recipes that call for minced beef by combining it with other meats. You get the flavour of beef yet reduced fat and cholesterol. Add a pound of drained, crumbled tofu to this recipe to extend it even further if you like, and adjust seasonings accordingly. These are delicious served over saffron or yellow rice, which you can find in your supermarket.

6 oz/175 g whole-wheat
  breadcrumbs
8 fl oz/225 ml skimmed milk
1½ lb/675 g minced turkey
8 oz/225 g extra lean minced beef
2 whole eggs
2 egg whites
1 large onion, finely chopped
1 scant teaspoon salt

½ teaspoon pepper
2 scant teaspoons sugar
½ teaspoon ginger
½ teaspoon nutmeg
½ teaspoon allspice
½ teaspoon dry mustard
1¼ pints/560 ml beef stock
3 tablespoons flour
1½ teaspoons instant coffee

1. Soak the breadcrumbs in the milk for several minutes.
2. Meanwhile, combine the minced turkey and beef.
3. Beat the whole eggs and egg whites together and add to the meat mixture. Add the moistened breadcrumbs, onion and season-ings to the meat mixture and mix well.

4. Form into 1½ inch/3 cm balls (makes 40–50) and refrigerate overnight.
5. Line up the meatballs on a large baking sheet (with edges) and cook in the oven at 350°F/Gas Mark 4/180°C for 25–30 minutes, turning halfway through cooking time.
6. While meatballs are cooking, heat stock in a large pot. Gradually add the flour, stirring constantly. Cook and stir until slightly thickened. Stir in the instant coffee.
7. Remove the meatballs from the oven and transfer them to the beef stock using a slotted spoon to allow grease to drain away. Simmer for 45 minutes and serve.

Makes 10 servings of 4 meatballs each.
Per serving: 313 calories, 122 mg cholesterol, 1 g dietary fibre, 14 g fat, 712 mg sodium

LAMB

Lamb, like pork, is a fatty meat that requires careful trimming to meet T-Factor guidelines. The recipe that follows shows how to serve lamb in combination with high-fibre, low-fat foods so that you end up with a meal that's relatively low in fat.

Curried Lamb with Vegetables

4 lamb loin or shoulder chops, about ¾ inch/2 cm thick
2 cloves garlic, minced
1 dessertspoon vegetable oil
8 fl oz/225 ml water or low-salt stock
1 scant teaspoon cumin
½ teaspoon ground ginger
¼ teaspoon ground coriander

¼ teaspoon cayenne pepper
½ teaspoon ground turmeric
1 medium courgette, cut into chunks
2 medium carrots, sliced
1 medium onion, cut in chunks
fresh-ground black pepper to taste
10 oz/300 g frozen peas

1. Trim any visible fat from chops, and brown with the garlic in the vegetable oil in a large lidded frying pan.
2. Remove the lamb and add the remaining ingredients except for the peas. Cover and bring to a boil. Reduce heat to simmer, and put the lamb back in the pan. Cover, and simmer for 30 minutes.
3. Add the peas, and simmer another 10 minutes, until vegetables are tender and lamb is cooked.

Makes 4 servings
Per serving: 223 calories, 60 mg cholesterol, 10 g dietary fibre, 10 g fat, 120 mg sodium

PORK

Although pork is not a mainstay of my diet, some cuts can be lean. The shoulder or sirloin runs to about 30 to 35 per cent fat. If the pork is combined with vegetable side-dishes, fresh salad, and whole-grain bread, or used in an Oriental-style main dish, the percentage of fat for the whole meal can be reduced considerably. Be sure to trim away all visible fat, however.

Bacon, on the other hand, is much higher in fat (65 per cent, calories and sodium. If you just can't bear to live completely without it, try substituting lean ham (about 33 per cent fat) in recipes that call for bacon. (We have just heard of a 'turkey bacon' that our informant said was very good, but we have not tried it. It is only 5 per cent fat per ounce.)

*Pork Tenderloin with Orange Marmalade

1 pork tenderloin (1 lb/450 g)	pinch of black pepper
1 tablespoon grainy coarse prepared mustard	3 tablespoons low-sugar orange marmalade
1 clove garlic, minced	4 fl oz/110 ml water
¼ teaspoon fresh rosemary, finely chopped	4 tablespoons chicken stock

1. Preheat oven to 400°F/Gas Mark 6/200°C. Make a cut lengthwise down the centre about halfway through the pork tenderloin.
2. In a small bowl mix together mustard, garlic, rosemary and black pepper. Spread mixture along the cut surface of the tenderloin. Reshape and tie in several places. Place on rack above roasting pan. Brush with half the marmalade. Add water to pan.
3. Bake in a preheated oven for 40 to 45 minutes. If you have a meat thermometer, the internal temperature should reach 160°F/71°C.
4. Mix together remaining orange marmalade and chicken stock in a small saucepan. Simmer 2 to 3 minutes until thickened. Spoon sauce over sliced tenderloin and serve immediately.

Makes 4 servings.
Per serving: 160 calories, 74 mg cholesterol, 0 dietary fibre, 3 g fat, 174 mg sodium

*Pork Chops Parmesan

2 tablespoons maizemeal, whole-wheat flour or breadcrumbs
1 dessertspoon grated Parmesan cheese
½ teaspoon fresh-ground black pepper
½ teaspoon salt
½ teaspoon basil
4 pork loin rib chops, about ½ inch/1 cm thick
1 dessertspoon vegetable oil
3 spring onions, chopped
1 clove garlic, minced
¼ teaspoon fennel seeds, crushed

1. Combine the maize meal, Parmesan cheese, black pepper, salt and basil.
2. Trim the pork chop of all visible fat, pat them dry and dredge in the meal mixture.
3. Heat a frying pan over medium heat, and add the oil. When the oil is hot, place the chops in the pan and reduce the heat to low.
4. Fry the chops for 10 minutes on each side. Then add the onions, garlic and fennel, and continue frying for another 10 minutes, turning as necessary to keep from sticking.

Makes 4 servings.
Per serving: 198 calories, 56 mg cholesterol, 1 g dietary fibre, 12 g fat, 340 mg sodium

Stir-Fry Pork with Mange Tout

4 pork chops
1 dessertspoon groundnut or vegetable oil
¼ teaspoon black pepper
1 dessertspoon soy sauce
1 clove garlic, crushed
1 slice fresh ginger, about ½ inch/1 cm thick, minced
1½ teaspoons sesame seeds
5 tablespoons water
4 spring onions or 1 leek, diced
6 oz/175 g fresh or frozen mange tout peas

1. Trim all visible fat from the chops, and slice the meat into thin strips, about ¼ inch/½ cm thick, and ½ to 1 inch/1–3 cm wide.
2. Heat the oil in a wok or large frying pan over medium heat, then add the pork and brown, stirring often.
3. Mix together the black pepper, soy sauce, garlic, ginger, sesame seeds and water, and add to the browned meat. Add the onions.
4. Cover, reduce heat, and let simmer for about 30 minutes, until the pork is cooked through, stirring occasionally. Add more water if necessary to prevent sticking.

5. Meanwhile, cook the mange tout without added salt. Add the cooked mange tout to the pork, stir, and serve.

Makes 4 servings.
Per serving: 237 calories, 55 mg cholesterol, 2 g dietary fibre, 14 g fat, 316 mg sodium

POULTRY

In comparison with red meats, chicken is a low-fat source of protein. A cooked half breast of chicken, about 3 oz/80 g of white meat *without skin*, averages around 140 calories. Only about 20 per cent of its nutrient weight, or 27 calories, comes from fat. Compare this to a *small* steak of around 3½ oz/95 g cooked, which could contain as much as 440 calories, with 360 of those calories coming from fat. You can see that, as a rule, chicken is the choice to make.

White chicken meat contains about 25 per cent less fat than dark meat. When whole chickens are used, the nutritional analyses assume half white meat, half dark. When a recipe calls for chicken breasts, split breasts are assumed; that is, 4 chicken breasts means 4 half breasts.

Turkey is also a low-fat favourite. Turkey mince is an excellent 'extender' for minced beef, or it can be used instead of minced beef in most recipes.

*Baked Chicken with Tarragon and Fennel

4 chicken breasts, skinned
1 scant teaspoon tarragon
¼ teaspoon fennel seeds, crushed
⅛ teaspoon cardamom
salt and fresh-ground black pepper to taste

1. Place chicken breasts on foil-lined baking tin. Sprinkle with seasonings. Cover loosely with foil to help retain moisture.
2. Bake at 350°F/Gas Mark 4/180°C for 45 to 50 minutes, until cooked through.

Makes 4 servings
Per serving: 165 calories, 84 mg cholesterol, 0 dietary fibre, 3.5 g fat, 207 mg sodium

*Baked Turkey Loaf

1½ lb/675 g minced turkey
½ medium onion, finely chopped
1 stalk celery, finely chopped
3 tablespoons fresh parsley, chopped
small piece sweet pepper, finely chopped
whole-wheat breadcrumbs from 2 large slices, toasted
3 tablespoons skimmed milk or chicken stock
1 egg white, slightly beaten
¼ teaspoon fresh-ground black pepper
¼ teaspoon dried oregano, crushed
1 clove garlic, crushed

1. Mix all ingredients until just blended. Do not overmix.
2. Press the mixture into a 4 × 9 inch/10 × 23 cm non-stick loaf-tin.
3. Bake at 325°F/Gas Mark 4/180°C for 45 minutes to 1 hour. Serve hot with Mushroom Glaze (page 152) or serve cold.

Makes 6 servings.
Per serving: 237 calories, 72 mg cholesterol, 1 g dietary fibre, 11.5 g fat, 179 mg sodium

Barbecued Chicken

You can use this recipe with our Barbecue Sauce (page 151) or your own variation.

3½ lb/1.6 kg chicken pieces   8 fl oz/225 ml barbecue sauce

1. Preheat oven to 350°F/Gas Mark 4/180°C.
2. Skin the chicken pieces. Place the pieces 'skin' side down in a large, shallow baking tin. (You may wish to line the tin with foil for easy cleaning.)
3. Baste the chicken pieces liberally with barbecue sauce, and place in the oven.
4. Bake at 350°F/Gas Mark 4/180°C for 20 minutes, basting halfway through. Then turn the chicken pieces over and bake another 25 to 30 minutes, or until chicken is tender, basting occasionally.

Makes 6 servings.
Per serving: 174 calories, 78 mg cholesterol, 1 g dietary fibre, 5 g fat, 86 mg sodium (analyses include Barbecue Sauce recipe)

Five-Pepper Fajitas

You may be able to buy ready-prepared salsa from a specialist shop or you can make your own (see Mexican-Style Hot Sauce, page 104). Fajitas ('little bundles' of various ingredients) can be messy if you eat them the traditional way in your hands, so you may want to use a knife and fork.

4 chicken breasts, skinned,   ½ teaspoon cumin
  boned   1 medium red pepper
juice of 1 lime   1 medium yellow pepper
2 cloves garlic, crushed   1 medium green pepper
4 spring onions, chopped   8 whole-wheat tortillas
fresh-ground black pepper to taste 1 dessertspoon vegetable oil

1 dessertspoon water
1–2 teaspoons jalapeño peppers, chopped fine
salt taste

fresh parsley, chopped, to taste
1 medium tomato, diced
salsa to taste

1. Slice the chicken into chunks about ½ inch/1 cm square. Place the pieces in a large bowl. Squeeze the lime juice over chicken. Add the garlic, onions, black pepper and cumin, and toss to mix.
2. Slice the peppers into strips and set aside.
3. Wrap the tortillas in a clean tea-towel, place them on an oven-proof plate and put the plate in the oven. Warm the tortillas at the lowest setting on your oven while preparing the fajita mixture.
4. Heat the oil and water in a large saucepan over medium heat and add the chicken, sweet peppers and jalapeño. Add the great amount of jalapeño if you like your food very spicy. Sauté, stirring frequently, until the chicken and vegetables are cooked through, about 25 minutes. Add salt to taste.
5. Spread a spoonful of the fajita mixture in a thick line in the middle of each tortilla. Top with parsley, tomato and salsa to taste. Roll up the tortillas and serve.

Makes 4 servings of 2 fajitas each
Per serving (2 fajitas): 421 calories, 84 mg cholesterol, 3 g dietary fat, 13 g fat, 508 mg sodium

Light and Easy Lemon Chicken

4 chicken breasts, skinned
1 scant teaspoon dried tarragon
2 lemons

fresh ground black pepper to
  taste

1. Remove all visible fat from chicken. Place each breast in the centre of a 12-inch/30-cm-square piece of aluminium foil. Fold the sides of the foil up so the lemon juice won't run out.
2. Halve the lemons and squeeze the juice of ½ lemon over each chicken breast. Sprinkle each breast with ¼ teaspoon of tarragon and the black pepper.
3. Fold the foil together and seal well to secure the chicken inside.
4. Place the wrapped chicken in a shallow baking dish and bake at 350°F/Gas Mark 4/180°C for about 45 minutes.

Makes 4 servings.
Per serving: 166 calories, 84 mg cholesterol, 0 dietary fibre, 3.5 g fat, 74 mg sodium

Marinade for Chicken Breasts

4 fl oz/110 ml wine (red or white)
1 scant teaspoon soy sauce

1 scant teaspoon ground ginger
1 dessertspoon lemon juice
2 spring onions, chopped

1. Combine ingredients. Remove the skin from chicken breasts and marinate for several hours, turning occasionally.
2. As you grill the chicken, baste it ocasionally with the marinade to prevent dryness.

Total per recipe: 90 calories, 0 cholesterol, 0 dietary fibre, 0 fat, 349 mg sodium

Quick Turkey Chop Suey

1 lb/450 g turkey mince
16 oz/450 g tin bean sprouts, drained
3 stalks celery, chopped
1 onion, chopped
8 oz/225 g tin water chestnuts, drained and sliced
5 oz/145 g tin sliced mushrooms, drained

¼ teaspoon ground ginger
10½ oz/315 g tin condensed beef or chicken consommé
2 dessertspoons soy sauce
2 dessertspoons cornflour
8 fl oz/225 ml measure of brown rice cooked in 16 fl oz/450 ml water

1. In a large frying pan, brown the ground turkey. Drain off any fat.
2. Add the vegetables, ginger and most of the consommé. Bring to a boil over medium-high heat. Reduce heat, cover, and simmer 20 minutes.
3. Combine the reserved consommé with the soy sauce and cornflour. Add to the meat and vegetable mixture, stirring until thickened and bubbly. Serve over the rice.

Makes 6 servings.
Per serving: 294 calories, 48 mg cholesterol, 4 g dietary fibre, 8 g fat, 679 mg sodium

MEATLESS MAIN COURSES

I usually have at least one meat-free day a week, when my breakfasts and lunches centre on dairy foods, vegetables and fruits, and my main course at dinner consists of protein-rich beans and rice or some other meatless dish. Many people in the Western world eat twice as much protein as they need each day, the majority of it coming from meat, which is higher in fat, cholesterol, chemical additives and cost than protein foods from the plant world.

Combinations of legumes, grains and seeds provide the same quality of protein as animal protein. Enhance them with dairy products or small amounts of meat if desired.

If you're used to eating a good hunk of meat for dinner each night, try some of these meatless meals for a change, and discover how satisfying they can be.

COOKING WHOLE GRAINS

To cook whole grains such as brown rice, you need about twice as much liquid (water or stock) as grain. Simply bring the liquid to a boil, add the rinsed grain, bring to a boil again, cover, reduce heat and let simmer for about 40 minutes. Stirring is unnecessary. Especially when cooked in stock, no added fat is needed to make whole grains taste good. You can always add herbs and spices or grated vegetables such as shallots or carrots if you want more flavour.

TOASTING SEEDS AND NUTS

To toast seeds or nuts without added fat, my favourite method is to put them in a dry frying pan over medium heat and brown them, stirring frequently.

Basic Better Beans

The use of stock instead of water for soaking and cooking, along with a whole onion stuck with whole cloves, makes beans even more flavourful. Serve with cooked grain for a main course.

16 fl oz/450 ml measure of dried beans or lentils (your choice)
1½ pints/850 ml chicken stock

2 large onions
6 whole cloves
2 dessertspoons olive oil
dash of salt and pepper

1. Soak the beans in the stock, together with the onions stuck with the cloves, overnight in the refrigerator. Lentils do not require soaking.

2. Remove the onions and cloves (discard cloves), and cook the plumped beans in the stock until just tender.
3. Chop the onions and sauté in the oil until translucent.
4. Place all ingredients (except cloves) in a large casserole dish and bake for 1 hour at 325°F/Gas Mark 3/170°C.

Makes 8 servings.
Per serving: 181 calories, 0 cholesterol, 6 g dietary fibre, 5 g fat, 438 mg sodium

Bean-and-Corn Chilli over Puffed Tortilla

Check package ingredients for tortillas made with no lard.

4 soft flour tortillas (7 inches/ 18 cm in diameter)
2 onions chopped
2 cloves of garlic, finely chopped
½ teaspoon of vegetable oil
1 tin (14 oz/400 g) of Italian-style plum tomatoes, drained
½ teaspoon of ground cumin
2 turns of fresh ground black pepper
pinch of red pepper flakes

1 tin (15¼ oz/430 g) of kidney beans (reserve 4 tablespoons of liquid)
1 tin (4 oz/110 g) of chopped mild green chillies, drained, or ½ teaspoon of fresh jalapeño pepper
8 oz/225 g of frozen whole-kernel sweetcorn, thawed
3 oz/85 g of low-fat Cheddar or other hard cheese

1. Arrange tortillas on foil-lined baking sheet. Watching carefully, bake tortillas at 450°F/Gas Mark 8/230°C for 4 to 5 minutes until puffed and lightly golden. Reserve.
2. Sauté onion and garlic in oil in a 12-inch/30 cm non-stick frying pan over medium heat for 3 to 4 minutes.
3. Add tomatoes, cumin, black pepper, red pepper, kidney beans and reserved liquid, and ½ of the green chillies. Simmer for 5 minutes, stirring often. Add sweetcorn and cook 1 minute longer.
4. Place a tortilla on each plate. Mound ¼ of the chilli mixture over each. Sprinkle each with ¼ of the cheese. Serve accompanied by the remaining green chillies.

Makes 4 servings.
Per serving: 305 calories, 15 mg cholesterol, 11 g dietary fibre, 8 g fat, 979 mg sodium. (If low-fat cheese is not available and you use ordinary Cheddar, add about 18 calories, 2 g fat, and 5 mg cholesterol per serving.)

*Aubergine Parmesan

Aubergine is known for its ability to absorb huge quantities of oil. This 'no-fry' version of a delectable Italian dish eliminated almost all of the oil and therefore, compared with a popular recipe, 75 grams of fat and 675 calories *per serving*. Protein in this recipe comes from the egg, milk and cheese, along with the wheatgerm and breadcrumbs.

1 medium aubergine
1 egg or 2 egg whites
2 dessertspoons skimmed milk
3 tablespoons wheatgerm
6 tablespoons breadcrumbs

1 dessertspoon Parmesan cheese
16 fl oz/450 ml Real Italian
Tomato Sauce (p. 140)
6 oz/175 g low-fat mozzarella
cheese, grated

1. Peel the aubergine and cut it into 8 slices, ½ inch/1 cm thick.
2. Beat together the egg (or egg whites) and milk in a small, shallow bowl.
3. In another bowl, combine the wheatgerm, breadcrumbs and Parmesan cheese.
4. Lightly oil a foil-lined baking sheet. Dip the aubergine slices into the egg mixture, coating well. Then dip them into the breadcrumb mixture. Place the slices on the baking sheet, and bake at 350°F/Gas Mark 4/180°C for 15 minutes. Turn the slices over, and bake for 10 more minutes.
5. Make a layer of aubergine in a casserole dish, top with tomato sauce, them mozzarella cheese. Repeat the layers.
6. Bake covered at 350°F/Gas Mark 4/180°C for 25 minutes, then uncover and bake 15 minutes more.

Makes 4 servings.
Per serving: 256 calories, 81 mg cholesterol, 9 g dietary fibre, 8 g fat, 438 mg sodium

*Indian Spiced Beans

Delicious served with 1 dessertspoon of grated cheese per serving, a choice of chopped vegetables and salsa. Add a helping of cooked grain such as rice for a complete meal.

12 oz/350 g dried red or kidney
beans
1½ pints/850 ml stock
1 medium onion, sliced
1 medium tomato, chopped
1 clove garlic, chopped

2 dried red chillies
1 bay leaf
¼ teaspoon fresh ground black
pepper
¼ teaspoon ground cloves

Wash beans and remove any stones. Place all ingredients in a large saucepan. Bring to a boil and let boil for ten minutes, then reduce heat. Cover and cook for 4 hours on low heat.

Makes 4½ servings.
Per serving: 210 calories, 0 cholesterol, 14 g dietary fibre, 1 g fat, 230 mg sodium

Picadillo and Cornbread Wedges

Cornbread wedges:

3 oz/80 g yellow maizemeal	2 egg whites
4 tablespoons unsifted white flour	5 fl oz/145 ml buttermilk
1 teaspoon baking powder	2 dessertspoons vegetable oil

Picadillo

1 large sweet green pepper, halved, cored, seeded and cut into ½ inch/1 cm pieces	½ teaspoon reduced-calorie margarine
1 large sweet red pepper, halved, cored, seeded and cut into ½ inch/1 cm pieces	two 15 oz/425 g tins red kidney beans, undrained
1 medium onion, chopped	½–¾ teaspoon ground cumin
1 clove garlic, finely chopped	¼ teaspoon ground red pepper
	4 fl oz/110 ml tomato sauce
	3 tablespoons sultanas

1. *Prepare cornbread:* Preheat oven to 400°F/Gas Mark 6/200°C. Lightly oil an 8 × 1½ inch/20 × 30 cm non-stick round cake-tin.
2. Stir together maizemeal, flour and baking powder in a medium bowl until well mixed.
3. Lightly beat egg whites in a small bowl. Stir in the buttermilk and oil until well combined.
4. Pour the liquid ingredients all at once into the dry ingredients. Stir the mixture briskly with a fork until all the ingredients are just evenly moistened; do not overstir. The batter will be lumpy. Turn into prepared tin.
5. Bake at 400°F/Gas Mark 6/200°C for 18 to 20 minutes or until a wooden pick inserted into the centre comes out clean. Turn out onto wire rack to cool slightly. Cut cornbread into 4 wedges; put on plates.
6. *Prepare picadillo:* Sauté peppers, onion and garlic in margarine in a large non-stick frying pan for 5 to 8 minutes. Stir in kidney beans, cumin, red pepper, tomato sauce and sultanas. Cook to thicken slightly, about 10 to 12 minutes over medium-high heat. Mixture should be sloppy.

7. Pour sauce over cornbread, dividing equally. Serve immediately.

Makes 4 servings.
Per serving: 451 calories, 2 mg cholesterol, 17 g dietary fibre, 9 g fat, 994 mg sodium

Spinach Lasagne

1 medium onion, chopped
2 cloves garlic, minced
1 dessertspoon olive oil
about 2 tablespoons water
1 lb/450 g low-fat ricotta cheese
3 tablespoons grated Parmesan
  cheese
1½ lb/675 g fresh spinach,
  chopped or frozen equivalent
2 egg whites, beaten
¼ teaspoon pepper

2 tablespoons fresh chopped
  parsley
1 lb/450 g firm tofu, drained
  and crumbled
1 lb/450 g lasagne noodles,
  preferably wholewheat
6 oz/175 g low-fat mozzarella
  cheese, grated
2½ pints/1.3 litres Real Italian
  Tomato Sauce (p. 140)

1. Sauté the onion and garlic in the olive oil, adding water as needed to keep from sticking.
2. Combine the ricotta, tofu (if used), Parmesan, spinach, egg whites, black pepper, parsley and sautéed onion and garlic, mixing well.
3. Cook the lasagne according to package directions.
4. Lightly oil a 13 × 9 × 2 inch/33 × 23 × 5 cm casserole. Arrange a layer of cooked noodles on the bottom, top with ⅓ of the ricotta mixture, sprinkle with mozzarella, and spread with tomato sauce. Repeat layers twice more, ending with sauce.
5. Cover the dish with foil, crimping edges tightly. Bake at 350°F/ Gas Mark 4/180°C for 40 minutes, remove foil and bake 10–15 minutes more.

Makes 12 servings.
Per serving (minus tofu): 215 calories, 21 mg cholesterol, 3.5 g dietary fibre, 8 g fat, 918 mg sodium

Vegetable Stroganoff

This is good served over cooked pasta or grains such as bulghur
  wheat or rice.

10 oz/300 g mushrooms, sliced
2 medium onions, sliced
1 clove garlic, crushed
1 scant teaspoon vegetable oil
water as needed
3 tablespoons whole-wheat
  flour
6 fl oz/180 ml vegetable stock
3 tablespoons dry sherry
1 tablespoon Worcestershire
  sauce
¼ teaspoon marjoram

⅛ teaspoon chilli powder
⅛ teaspoon thyme
dash of nutmeg
fresh ground black pepper to
  taste
two 15 oz/425 g tins pinto
  beans or cooked equivalent
  (8 oz/225 g raw), drained
12 fl oz/330 ml plain low-fat
  yoghurt
1 teaspoon lemon juice

1. In a large lidded frying pan sauté/steam mushrooms, onions
   and garlic in the oil and a little water as needed.
2. In a bowl or measuring cup, mix together the flour, stock,
   sherry, Worcestershire sauce and seasonings.
3. When mushrooms are tender, stir in the stock mixture and cook
   until thickened, stirring occasionally.
4. Stir in the beans and heat through.
5. Remove from heat. Stir in the yoghurt and lemon juice and
   serve.

Makes 6 servings.
Per serving: 225 calories, 1 mg cholesterol, 11.5 g dietary fibre, 2 g
fat, 116 mg sodium

PASTA

High in carbohydrates and low in fat, pasta is one of my favourite T-Factor foods. Cook it *al dente*, not mushy, and enjoy it with some of the wonderful sauces presented here. Sample pastas made from different grains.

An average serving of cooked pasta contains about 2 grams of fat.

If you're watching your cholesterol intake, you can use cholesterol-free pasta made from enriched semolina rather than egg noodles, which contains about 50 milligrams of cholesterol per serving.

*Pasta and Shrimps with Ricotta Cheese Sauce

2 large cloves garlic, finely chopped
¼ teaspoon crushed red pepper flakes
1 scant teaspoon reduced-calorie margarine
4 fl oz/110 ml skimmed milk
6 oz/175 g low-fat ricotta
8 oz/225 g cooked shrimps, shelled and sliced horizontally
1 package (10 oz/300 g) frozen peas, thawed completely
2 tablespoons chopped parsley
½ teaspoon salt
⅛ teaspoon ground nutmeg
2–3 dashes Tabasco
3 tablespoons grated reduced-fat Cheddar-type cheese (1 oz/28 g)
12 oz/350 g linguine or other flat pasta

1. Sauté garlic and red pepper flakes in hot margarine in a 10 inch/25 cm non-stick frying pan for 2 minutes or until garlic is golden.
2. Whisk in milk and ricotta until smooth. Add shrimps, peas, parsley, salt, nutmeg and Tabasco and heat through.
3. Stir in grated cheese or reserve to sprinkle over later.
4. Meanwhile, cook pasta in a large pan of boiling water following package directions. Drain and rinse quickly in hot water. Transfer to large bowl.
5. Top pasta with hot sauce. Toss well to coat. Serve immediately.

Makes 6 servings.
Per serving: 357 calories, 113 mg cholesterol, 2 g dietary fibre, 7 g fat, 368 mg sodium

Hot Pasta Salad California

This makes a delightful main course for a light supper or special luncheon. It's also good served in smaller portions as a side dish.

2 scant teaspoons butter
2 medium yellow or green courgettes
2 teaspoons water
14 oz/400 g tin artichoke hearts, drained and rinsed

6 sprigs fresh parsley, chopped
dash of salt
3 tablespoons Parmesan cheese (optional)
8 oz/225 g dry vermicelli or other pasta, cooked

1. Melt butter over low heat in a large saucepan. Slice the courgettes into ⅛ to ¼ inch/¼ to ½ cm rounds. Add the courgettes and water to the butter. Cover and cook for 5 minutes, stirring occasionally.
2. Cut the artichoke hearts into quarters and stir into the courgettes along with the parsley and salt. Cover and heat through. Serve hot over hot cooked pasta. Sprinkle with Parmesan if desired.

Makes 4 servings as a main course.
Per serving (including 1 tablespoon Parmesan): 257 calories, 9 mg cholesterol, 6 g dietary fibre, 4.5 g fat, 311 mg sodium

*Scallop-and-Clam Pasta

1 dessertspoon of olive oil
2 dessertspoons of water
2 large white onions, sliced thin
8 to 10 cloves of garlic, minced
6 oz/175 g of fresh mushrooms, quartered
4 tins (6½ to 7 oz/190 to 200 g each) of clams, with their juice
1 oz/28 g of butter
2 dessertspoons of whole-wheat flour
2 tablespoons evaporated skimmed milk

3 fl oz/70 ml skimmed milk
2 dessertspoons dried skimmed milk
1 pound/450 g spaghetti
Water for cooking spaghetti
1 pound/450 g scallops, drained
3 tablespoons grated Parmesan cheese (1 oz/28 g in weight)
¼ teaspoon of cayenne (scant)
⅛ teaspoon of cloves
⅛ teaspoon of ginger
⅛ teaspoon of mace
Fresh-ground black pepper to taste

1. Heat the oil and water in a large saucepan. Add the onions, garlic, and mushrooms. Cover and let sauté/steam for a few minutes. Add the clams and their juice and let cook, covered.
2. In another pan, melt the butter. Blend in the whole-wheat flour,

stirring constantly, to form a roux. Add the evaporated milk, skimmed milk and dried milk. Pour the resulting sauce into the clam mixture.

3. In a large pot, heat the water to boiling. Add the spaghetti.
4. While the spaghetti is cooking, add the scallops to the clam sauce. Stir in the Parmesan cheese. Let simmer on very low heat for a few minutes, until the scallops are tenderly cooked. Stir in the seasonings and serve. You can add more Parmesan at the table, if desired.

Makes 10 servings.
Per serving: 258 calories, 85 mg cholesterol, 1 g dietary fibre, 9 g fat, 350 mg sodium

Red Clam Sauce

4 onions, chopped
12 oz/350 g of mushrooms, sliced
6 cloves of garlic, crushed
2 dessertspoons of olive oil
¼ teaspoon of salt
⅛ teaspoon of black pepper

pinch cayenne
1 tin (10½ oz/295 g) of tomato puree
4 tins (6½ oz/190 g each) of clams, minced with liquid

1. In a large saucepan, sauté onions, mushrooms, and garlic in the oil over medium-low heat for about 5 minutes, or until onions are translucent.
2. Add remaining ingredients and cook, covered, for 45 minutes.

Makes about 3 pints/1.7 litres (8 servings).
Per 8 fl oz/225 ml: 124 calories, 63 mg cholesterol, 2 g dietary fibre, 4.5 g fat, 185 mg sodium

*Meat Sauce

2 onions, sliced
8 oz/225 g mushrooms, sliced
3 cloves garlic, crushed
2 dessertspoons olive oil
1 lb/450 g lean mince
1 dessertspoon dried basil

6 oz/175 g tin tomato paste
28 oz/800 g tin whole tomatoes
½ teaspoon black pepper
½ teaspoon salt
¼ teaspoon cayenne or crushed red pepper

1. In a large saucepan, heat the oil and sauté the onion, mushrooms and garlic over medium-low heat for about 5 minutes or until onions are translucent.

139

2. Add mince and continue to cook for about 5 minutes or until beef is browned. Drain visible fat.
3. Add remaining ingredients and blend well together, breaking up the whole tomatoes with the spoon as you stir.
4. Cover the pan, reduce heat, and cook on low for 1 hour.

Serves 8.
Per serving: 198 calories, 37 mg cholesterol, 2.5 g dietary fibre, 12 g fat, 343 mg sodium

Real Italian Tomato Sauce

Here is our favourite basic standby sauce. It can be used for any recipe calling for tomato sauce, from pasta to fish. You can store it in a tightly sealed container in the refrigerator for up to a week, or freeze it for later use.

Look for no-salt-added tinned tomato products if you're trying to cut down on salt.

1 dessertspoon olive oil	1 large bay leaf
1 medium onion, cut in chunks	28 oz/800 g tin tomatoes
8 oz/225 g fresh mushrooms, sliced or quartered	11 oz/325 g tin tomato purée
1–2 tablespoons dried basil (even more if you use fresh!)	6 oz/175 g tin tomato paste
2 large cloves garlic, crushed or minced	salt and fresh-ground black pepper to taste

1. Heat a large saucepan over medium heat. Put in the oil, onion, mushrooms, basil and garlic. Cover, and reduce the heat to medium low. Stir frequently – you may need to add a tablespoon or two of water to keep it from sticking.
2. When the onions are translucent, add the remaining ingredients, except the salt and pepper. Bring to a boil on high heat, then reduce to simmer and let cook for an hour or so, stirring occasionally and breaking up the whole tomatoes.
3. Add salt and pepper to taste.

Makes about 2½ pints/1.3 litres (6 servings)
Per 8 fl oz/225 ml: 110 calories, 0 cholesterol, 4 g dietary fibre, 3 g fat, 326 mg sodium

VEGETABLE AND GRAIN SIDE-DISHES

Fresh raw or steamed vegetables are a low-fat complement to any meal. Cooked in a microwave, vegetables retain their nutrients perhaps better than through any other way of cooking. Check your microwave manual for the simple instructions for cooking vegetables.

Leave edible skins on most vegetables and fruits, such as apples, carrots and potatoes. The skins contain healthy nutrients and fibre.

Frozen vegetables are good to have on hand, but tinned ones are usually overcooked, over-salted or preserved with ingredients you may prefer to avoid, so read labels carefully.

Nutritionists now believe that we should eat a leafy green vegetable every day not only for the vitamin A content but also for the calcium. Many have almost the same amount of calcium as milk products, and no fat!

*Apple-Sweet Sweet Potatoes

3 large sweet potatoes
6 fl oz/175 ml water
3 medium apples, cored, peeled, sliced ½ inch/1 cm thick
8 fl oz/225 ml unsweetened apple juice

2 dessertspoons cornflour
3 dessertspoons unsweetened apple juice
1 dessertspoon honey
3 tablespoons wheatgerm
3 tablespoons toasted breadcrumbs

1. Cook whole sweet potatoes in water until tender, about 20 minutes. Peel and slice lengthwise about ½ inch/1 cm thick. Layer slices in a large casserole dish. Top with apple slices.
2. In a saucepan, bring 8 fl oz/225 ml of apple juice to a boil.
3. Dissolve the cornflour in the remaining apple juice and add to the hot juice. Stir until thickened. Stir in honey. Pour the sauce over the apples and sweet potatoes.
4. Combine the wheatgerm and breadcrumbs. Sprinkle on top of casserole.
5. Bake at 350°F/Gas Mark 4/180°C for 45 minutes or until apples are fork tender.

Makes 8 servings.
Per serving: 168 calories, 0 cholesterol, 4 g dietary fibre, 1 g fat, 34 mg sodium

Baby Carrots

1 lb/450 g whole baby carrots   ½ teaspoon Herb Salt (p. 153)
4 fl oz/110 ml water   pepper to taste
½ chicken bouillon cube

1. Trim stems from carrots and scrub.
2. Combine all ingredients in a casserole dish and bake at 350°F/ Gas Mark 4/180°C for about 45 minutes until carrots are tender.

Makes 4 servings.
Per serving: 52 calories, 0 cholesterol, 4 g dietary fibre, 0 fat, 646 mg sodium

Beetroot à l'Orange

3 dessertspoons grated orange   1 dessertspoon cornflour
   rind   2 lb/450 g beetroot, cooked and
8 fl oz/225 ml orange juice   sliced
½ teaspoon salt   fresh ground black pepper

1. Combine the orange rind, juice, salt and cornflour in the top of a double boiler. Cook and stir until thickened.
2. Add the beetroot and heat through. Sprinkle with black pepper.

Makes 6 servings.
Per serving: 61 calories, 0 cholesterol, 3 g dietary fibre, 0 fat, 234 mg sodium

Broccoli with Almonds

1½ teaspoons butter   chopped in florets, stems
2 dessertspoons almonds, chop-   diced
   ped or slivered   1 tablespoon water
2 large stalks fresh broccoli,

1. Melt the butter in a lidded frying pan over medium heat. Add the almonds and toast, stirring frequently, until browned, about 2 to 3 minutes.
2. Add the broccoli and stir to coat with the almonds.
3. Add the water, cover, and reduce heat to low. Sauté/steam for 10 to 15 minutes, until tender, stirring frequently and adding more water if necessary.

Makes 4 servings.
Per serving: 54 calories, 5 mg cholesterol, 2 g dietary fibre, 4 g fat, 27 mg sodium

*Brussels Sprouts with Caraway Seeds

1 lb/450 g Brussels sprouts
water or chicken stock
1 scant teaspoon caraway seeds

¼ teaspoon salt
¼ teaspoon pepper

1. Wash Brussels sprouts and trim wilted leaves. Make a gash in the bottom of each to speed cooking.
2. Place in 4 fl oz/110 ml of boiling water or stock. Reduce heat, cover and cook until fork tender. Do not overcook.
3. Pour off liquid. Add seeds and seasonings.

Makes 4 servings.
Per serving: 45 calories, 0 cholesterol, 3.5 g dietary fibre, 1 g fat, 233 mg sodium

Creamed Spinach and Turnip Tops

10 oz/300 g package chopped
  frozen spinach
10 oz/300 g turnip tops,
  chopped
1 dessertspoon butter
2 dessertspoons whole-wheat
  flour

8 fl oz/225 ml skimmed milk
2 scant teaspoons Herb Salt
  (p. 153)
garlic powder to taste
salt to taste
1 dessertspoon breadcrumbs

1. Cook turnip tops for 3 minutes in boiling water. Drain and combine with defrosted spinach in a casserole dish.
2. Melt butter in a saucepan and add flour gradually, stirring well. Add milk slowly, mixing constantly. Add seasonings (not crumbs) and heat until thickened. Pour over greens.
3. Top with crumbs and bake at 325°F/Gas Mark 3/170°C until bubbly, about 30 minutes.

Makes 8 servings.
Per serving: 53 calories, 4 mg cholesterol, 2.5 g dietary fibre, 2 g fat, 109 mg sodium

Green Beans Creole

1 lb/450 g fresh or frozen
  French beans
water
16 oz/450 g tin tomatoes
1 stalk celery, finely chopped

½ sweet pepper, chopped
½ teaspoon onion powder
dash of salt
dash of crushed red pepper
  (optional)

1. Trim beans if necessary and steam over water for 5 minutes, until just tender, or cook frozen beans as package directs.
2. Combine the cooked beans with the remaining ingredients in a large saucepan. Heat over medium heat for about 15 minutes or until all vegetables are tender.

Makes 8 servings.
Per serving: 30 calories, 0 cholesterol, 3 g dietary fibre, 0 fat, 140 mg sodium

Scalloped Potatoes

1 large onion, thinly sliced	½ teaspoon salt
1 dessertspoon butter	1 dessertspoon whole-wheat
2 large potatoes, thinly sliced	flour
2 dessertspoons lemon juice	2 dessertspoons breadcrumbs
1 scant teaspoon thyme	8 fl oz/225 ml skimmed milk

1. Sauté the onions in the butter until translucent. Add the potatoes and combine. Add the lemon juice, thyme and salt, and mix.
2. Lightly oil a casserole dish. Put half the potato mixture in the casserole and sprinkle with the flour. Add the rest of the potatoes. Pour in the skimmed milk, and sprinkle with the breadcrumbs.
3. Bake at 325°F/Gas Mark 3/170°C for 1 hour or until potatoes are tender and slightly browned on top.

Makes 4 servings.
Per serving: 187 calories, 9 mg cholesterol, 3 g dietary fibre, 3.5 g fat, 354 mg sodium

Scandinavian-Style Potato Casserole

1 oz/28 g butter	thinly as possible
2 oz/56 g tin anchovy fillets	¼ teaspoon salt
2 large onions, sliced as thinly as possible	fresh ground black pepper to taste
1 dessertspoon caraway seeds	8 fl oz/225 ml skimmed milk
2 lb/900 g baking potatoes (3–4 large), skins on, sliced as	8 oz/225 g low-fat cheese

1. Melt most of the butter in a large frying pan over medium heat. Drain the anchovies, rinse them in a strainer and chop them.

Add the anchovies, onions and caraway seeds to the butter and cook just until the onions are soft, about 10 minutes.

2. Combine the potatoes and the onion mixture, tossing to mix. Pour the mixture into a large shallow baking dish. Sprinkle salt and pepper over the top.

3. In a bowl, blend together the milk and ricotta cheese with a wire whisk. Pour this mixture over the potatoes; it will still be a little lumpy, but that's okay. Dot with the remaining butter.

4. Bake at 400°F/Gas Mark 6/200°C for 1 hour, or until top is nicely browned.

Makes 12 servings.
Per serving: 157 calories, 16 mg cholesterol, 2 g dietary fibre, 4.5 g fat, 107 mg sodium

Courgette Mushroom Mix (Microwave)

2 onions, chopped
1 dessertspoon oil
2 dessertspoons water
2 lb/900 g courgettes, cut in ½ inch/1 cm chunks (use half yellow and half green courgettes if possible)

⅛ teaspoon thyme
fresh-ground black pepper to taste
8 oz/225 g fresh mushrooms, sliced thickly

1. Sauté onions in oil and water for about 7 minutes on high in the microwave, until the onions are translucent.

2. Add the courgettes, thyme and black pepper and microwave on high for about 12 minutes, until vegetables are just tender, stirring half-way through the cooking time.

3. Add the mushrooms and cook 2 to 3 minutes more on high until the mushrooms are tender. Add more water in small amounts if necessary during cooking.

Makes 10 servings.
Per serving: 37 calories, 0 cholesterol, 2 g dietary fibre, 1.5 g fat, 3 mg sodium

SALADS

Nutritionists recommend that about half the vegetables we eat each day should be raw. Uncooked vegetables are higher in fibre and nutrients than their cooked counterparts. In addition to fresh fruit, raw vegetables in a salad or alone make a great crunchy very low fat snack.

Bulghur Salad with Sunflower Seeds

Bulghur is a cracked wheat used most often in Middle Eastern cuisine. Rather than cooking it, soak it in water as directed below, and you will have a tender, fluffy grain. You can actually use any of your favourite fresh vegetables with any cooked grain to make an interesting meal-in-one luncheon salad such as this. You can even toss in some left-over cooked greens or other cooked vegetables.

8 fl oz/225 ml measure of
  bulghur wheat
16 fl oz/450 ml water, boiling
  hot
2 large tomatoes, diced
1 medium cucumber, diced
1 courgette, diced
2 spring onions, chopped fine
1 dessertspoon dried parsley (or
  3 dessertspoons fresh)
3 tablespoons dry-roasted
  unsalted sunflower seeds

The dressing:
1 scant teaspoon oregano
1 scant teaspoon soy sauce
½ teaspoon salt
1 scant teaspoon black pepper
1 dessertspoon olive oil
2 dessertspoons lemon juice
1 dessertspoon water

1. Soak the bulghur wheat in a bowl in the boiling water for 15 minutes. The wheat will soak up the water and become puffy and chewable. Drain any excess water if necessary.
2. In the meantime, combine all dressing ingredients.
3. When the wheat is ready, add the chopped vegetables, parsley and sunflower seeds, mixing well, then add the dressing. Toss and serve.

Makes 4 servings.
Per serving: 263 calories, 0 cholesterol, 8 g dietary fibre, 8.5 g fat, 363 mg sodium

Pink Potato Salad

4 oz/110 g cooked beetroot, diced
4 large potatoes, skins on, diced
½ green pepper, diced
4 fl oz/110 ml plain very low fat
  yoghurt

2 tablespoons mayonnaise
2 hard-boiled eggs, diced
salt, pepper, garlic and onion
  powder to taste

1. Boil the potatoes in a small amount of water until tender. Drain.
2. Combine with remaining ingredients in a large bowl. Chill before
   serving.

Makes about 8 servings.
Per serving: 155 calories, 72 mg cholesterol, 2 g dietary fibre, 5.5 g fat,
161 mg sodium

Spinach Salad Parmesan

1 lb/450 g fresh spinach leaves,
  washed well and trimmed
½ sweet red onion, thinly sliced
1 lb/450 g cherry tomatoes
4 oz/110 g fresh mushrooms,
  sliced

6 radishes, thinly sliced
1 dessertspoon grated Parmesan
  cheese

Toss together all ingredients. Serve with your favourite no- or low-fat
dressing.

Makes about 6 servings.
Per serving: 36 calories, 1 mg cholesterol, 4 g dietary fibre, 1 g fat, 60 mg
sodium (analyses are for no-fat dressing)

Sweet 'n' Savoury Chicken Salad

4 fl oz/110 ml very low fat
  yoghurt
1 dessertspoon lemon juice
½ teaspoon dried tarragon,
  crushed
about 1 lb/450 g cooked chicken,
  cut in chunks
20 oz/560 g tin pineapple
  chunks, unsweetened, drained

10½ oz/315 g tin mandarin
  oranges, unsweetened, drained
4 oz/110 g tin water chestnuts,
  drained and sliced
1 small cucumber, diced
2 spring onions, finely chopped
lettuce leaves

1. Mix together the yoghurt, lemon juice and tarragon to make a dressing.
2. In a large bowl, combine the remaining ingredients except the lettuce leaves. Pour the dressing over the chicken salad and toss lightly. Serve on lettuce leaves of your choice.

Makes 6 servings.
Per serving: 195 calories, 40 mg cholesterol, 2.5 g dietary fibre, 2 g fat, 57 mg sodium

SALAD DRESSINGS

Many people go to the salad bar in a restaurant, load their tray with vegetables and fruits, and congratulate themselves on their low-fat choice. At the same time, though, they often take several table-spoonfuls of high-fat salad dressings, adding several hundred calories and many grams of fat to an otherwise healthy meal.

Included here are three no-fat and two low-fat dressings. Creamy dressings usually have a base of plain, very low fat yoghurt, while the oil-and-vinegar varieties are 'stretched' with the addition of water.

Olive oil is a wonderful base for dressings, especially because it is a mono-unsaturated fat. Studies have shown that such fats (olive, groundnut, avocado) in reasonable amounts may have the effect of reducing cholesterol.

Balsamic Dressing

If you don't have balsamic vinegar, you may substitute another kind. But in that case, start with water and vinegar in equal proportions.

6 fl oz/175 ml water
2 fl oz/50 ml balsamic vinegar
2 teaspoons capers
1½ teaspoons Dijon mustard

1 teaspoon dried basil
1 tablespoon fresh parsley, chopped (optional)

Combine the ingredients. Adjust vinegar to taste, since it has a strong flavour. Store in a covered container in the refrigerator.

Makes about 8 fl oz/225 ml.
Per dessertspoon: 1 calorie, 0 cholesterol, 9 dietary fibre, 0 fat, 7 mg sodium

Creamy Dijon Dressing

4 fl oz/110 ml very low fat plain yoghurt
1 teaspoon Dijon mustard
1½ tablespoons grated cucumber

1 small spring onion, minced
2 teaspoons fresh parsley, chopped
dash of fresh ground black pepper

Combine all ingredients, mixing well. Serve chilled over your favourite salad greens and vegetables.

Makes about 4 fl oz/110 ml.
Per 2 dessertspoons: 19 calories, 1 mg cholesterol, 0 dietary fibre, 0 fat, 47 mg sodium

No-Fat Italian Dressing

3 tablespoons lemon juice
3 tablespoons cider vinegar
3 tablespoons unsweetened
  apple juice
½ teaspoon oregano
½ teaspoon dry mustard

½ teaspoon onion powder
1 clove garlic, cut in half
½ teaspoon paprika
¼ teaspoon basil
⅛ teaspoon thyme
⅛ teaspoon rosemary

Combine all ingredients. Chill for an hour or two at least to allow herbs to blend. Remove garlic clove pieces before serving.

Per 2 dessertspoons: 9 calories, 0 cholesterol, 9 dietary fibre, 0 fat, 1 mg sodium

*Sweet Yoghurt Dressing

With this fresh chopped fruit becomes a special light dessert.

8 fl oz/225 ml very low fat plain
  yoghurt
3 tablespoons golden raisins or
  sultanas

3 tablespoons chopped nuts
  (walnuts or other)
1 tablespoon honey

Mix all ingredients and chill overnight. Serve cold.

Makes about 12 fl oz/330 ml.
Per 2 dessertspoons: 45 calories, 0 cholesterol, 0.5 g dietary fibre, 1.5 g fat, 15 mg sodium

Tarragon–Dijon Dressing

1 dessertspoon olive oil
3 tablespoons red wine vinegar
2 dessertspoons lemon juice
4 tablespoons water
1 scant teaspoon prepared
  Dijon mustard
1 teaspoon tarragon, crushed

1 garlic clove, crushed
1 shallot or 2 spring onions,
  finely minced
1 dessertspoon honey
¼ teaspoon paprika
fresh-ground black pepper and
  salt to taste

Combine all ingredients well. Store in refrigerator.

Makes about 8 fl oz/225 ml.
Per 2 dessertspoons: 27 calories, 0 cholesterol, 0 dietary fibre, 2 g fat, 9 mg sodium

SAUCES

Traditional sauces are usually bursting with butter or other fats. Here you will find examples of tasty sauces to accompany your meals that can be made with little or no fat.

*Barbecue Sauce

This sauce will keep for about 10 days in the refrigerator.

12 oz/430 g tin no-salt-added tomato paste
3 tablespoons dry red wine (or substitute water)
12 fl oz/570 ml water or stock
2 dessertspoons red wine vinegar
2 teaspoons lemon juice
½ medium onion, chopped fine
½ medium sweet pepper, chopped fine
1 dessertspoon Worcestershire sauce

2 dessertspoons brown sugar
1 dessertspoon honey
1½ teaspoons liquid smoke
1 scant teaspoon garlic powder
1 dessertspoon chilli powder
1 dessertspoon dry mustard
crushed red pepper to taste
dash of Tabasco
2 tablespoons fresh parsley, minced
¼ teaspoon celery seed
½ teaspoon salt (optional)

1. Combine all ingredients except parsley and celery seed (and salt, if you're using any) in a large saucepan. Bring to a low boil, then reduce heat and simmer about 20 minutes.
2. Add the parsley, celery seed and salt (if desired), and simmer for another 5 minutes or so.

Makes about 1½ pints/1 litre.
Per dessertspoon: 8 calories, 0 cholesterol, 0 dietary fibre, 0 fat, 5 mg sodium

Light Béarnaise Sauce

3 tablespoons chicken or vegetable stock
3 tablespoons flour or 2 dessertspoons cornflour
16 fl oz/450 ml skimmed milk
2 oz/56 g dried skimmed milk

1 bay leaf
½ teaspoon thyme
½ teaspoon white pepper
1 scant teaspoon vegetable seasoning (optional)

151

1. Heat chicken or vegetable stock over moderate heat in a saucepan.
2. Gradually add flour or cornflour and blend with a wire whisk or wooden spoon.
3. Simmer and stir until heated through but not browned.
4. Remove from heat and add remaining ingredients.
5. Return to heat and cook, stirring occasionally, until thickened.

Makes 2 pints/900 ml.
Per 3 tablespoons: 42 calories, 1 mg cholesterol, 0 dietary fibre, 0 fat, 63 mg sodium (without optional vegetable seasoning; however, a salt-free vegetable seasoning will add no sodium)

*Mushroom Glaze

6 oz/175 g fresh mushrooms (leave whole if small, otherwise slice)

12 fl oz/330 ml chicken stock
2 dessertspoons cornflour
1–2 tablespoons cold water

1. Simmer mushrooms in chicken stock for 7 minutes.
2. Add cornflour to water and mix to a smooth paste. Gradually add the paste to the hot mushroom mixture and cook, stirring occasionally, until thickened.

Makes 12 fl oz/330 ml.
Per 2 dessertspoons: 8 calories, 0 cholesterol, 0 dietary fibre, 0 fat, 0 sodium (unless using tinned consommé which would be 32 mg sodium)

'Sour Cream' Topping

Vary this topping endlessly by substituting different herbs and spices for the chives listed below.

6 oz/175 g low-fat cottage cheese
3 dessertspoons skimmed milk

2 teaspoons lemon juice
chives to taste

Combine all ingredients in a blender or food processor and whir until smooth.

Makes about 8 fl oz/225 ml.
Per 3 tablespoons: 35 calories, 2 mg cholesterol, 0 dietary fibre, 0.5 g fat, 178 mg sodium

SEASONINGS

'Salt to taste' can be a dangerous instruction in the hands of some people. Human taste buds adapt to the tastes of salt and sugar, so that the more we use, the less sensitive to the flavour we become.

Although sodium (which comprises 40 per cent of table salt, the other 60 per cent being chloride) is an essential nutrient, many people in the Western world consume about eight to ten times more than their bodies need to stay healthy. Many of us are 'salt sensitive' and can develop high blood pressure in response to this over-consumption. Therefore, most health professionals, myself included, recommend cutting back on salt. Add less salt in cooking and eat fewer processed meats, soups and snack foods. It isn't necessary to cut out table salt completely, however, unless your doctor recommends a severely salt-restricted diet. Salt does seem to bring out the flavour in other foods, so many of the recipes in this book do use *small* amounts of it. When a recipe says 'salt to taste,' go lightly. Let other people add more salt at the table if they wish.

Perhaps the best way to reduce your use of salt is to gradually add less to your food over a period of a couple of weeks, and learn to use herbs and spices. Try some of the seasoning mixtures presented here, and then experiment with your own. Keep a wide variety on hand to inspire your creativity in the kitchen. Some commercially prepared sodium-free herb combinations may also appeal to your taste buds. Avoid garlic and onion salts, as they have far more sodium than plain garlic and onion powders. Herbs and spices are a real boon for people on a low-fat diet who miss the flavour of fat.

By the way, fresh herbs are less potent than equivalent amounts of dried, so triple the amount called for if substituting fresh for dried.

Herb Salt

This is one of my favourite combinations of herbs. Experiment with your own favourites as well. You will soon find that a herb salt is an excellent substitute for plain salt, and instead of about 2,000 to 2,200 milligrams of sodium per scant teaspoon it has only 285 milligrams.

½ teaspoon basil	¼ teaspoon celery seed
¼ teaspoon thyme	¼ teaspoon salt
¼ teaspoon dill weed	¼ teaspoon dried parsley

Combine all ingredients and grind with a mortar and pestle. Store in a small herb jar.

Makes about 1¾ teaspoons.
Except for the sodium mentioned above, the mixture contains only trace amounts of other nutrients too small to evaluate.

DESSERTS

Yes, you can have your cake and eat it too! If as a rule you follow the guidelines of the T-Factor Diet, there is room for an occasional pudding or cake, especially a comparatively low-fat one such as those in this section.

You can adapt many of your own favourite recipes as well to lower fat, more healthy versions. Substitute whole-wheat flour for at least part of the refined white flour, for higher fibre and higher nutrient content. Use fresh and dried fruits for sweetness and reduce refined sugar. Instead of making fatty pastry crusts with lard, butter, or vegetable shortening, learn to make crumb crusts with very little fat and honey, as in the scrumptious Pumpkin Cheesecake (page 158) and Chocolate Meringue Pie (below). The use of low-fat dairy products instead of their high-fat counterparts (skimmed milk instead of whole milk or cream, ricotta instead of cream cheese, for example) can reduce fat content considerably.

Of course, 'moderation' is a key concept when it comes to sweets that also contain fat. With this in mind, you can enjoy a treat now and then without destroying your waistline or your arteries.

*Chocolate Meringue Pie

12 fl oz/330 ml measure plain biscuit crumbs (about 6 oz/175 g)
2 dessertspoons runny honey
1 dessertspoon oil
6 oz/175 g sugar
4 tablespoons cocoa powder
3 dessertspoons cornflour
¼ teaspoon salt
16 fl oz/450 ml skimmed milk
1 egg, beaten
1 teaspoon vanilla essence
3 egg whites
¼ teaspoon cream of tartar
¼ teaspoon vanilla essence
4 tablespoons sugar

1. Combine the biscuit crumbs, honey and oil. Mix well and press into a 9 inch/23 cm flan-tin. Bake for 10 minutes at 350°F/Gas Mark 4/180°C.
2. Meanwhile, in a medium saucepan, combine the 6 oz/175 g of sugar, cocoa powder, flour and salt. Place over moderate heat and gradually stir in milk. Cook and stir until thickened and bubbly. Continue to cook 1 to 2 more minutes.
3. Remove from heat. Stir a small amount of the hot mixture into the beaten egg. Add egg to saucepan, return to heat, and cook 2 more minutes.
4. Stir in the 1 teaspoon of vanilla essence. Pour the mixture into the prepared crust.

5. To make topping, beat egg whites with cream of tartar and ½ teaspoon of vanilla until the mixture forms soft peaks. Gradually add the 6 tablespoons of sugar, beating until glossy and the mixture forms stiff peaks.
6. Spread the topping over the filling. Bake at 350°F/Gas Mark 4/180°C until golden brown, about 12 minutes.

Makes 8 servings.
Per serving: 295 calories, 35 mg cholesterol, 2.5 g dietary fibre, 5.5 g fat, 265 mg sodium: approx. figures as the fat and sugar content of biscuits varies. Check the packet for the lowest suitable kind.

Cocoa Pudding Cake

4 oz/110 g plain white flour
5 oz/145 g sugar
2 dessertspoons cocoa powder
1½ teaspoons baking powder
½ teaspoon salt
4 fl oz/110 ml skimmed milk

2 dessertspoons oil
½ teaspoon vanilla essence
5 oz/145 g soft brown sugar
3 level tablespoons cocoa powder
14 fl oz/380 ml hot water

1. Sift together the flour, 6 oz/175 g sugar, 2 dessertspoons of cocoa powder, baking powder and salt.
2. Add the milk, oil and vanilla, stirring until smooth.
3. Pour into a baking tin at least 8 × 8 × 2 inches/20 × 20 × 5 cm that has been lightly oiled.
4. Combine the brown sugar, ¼ cup of cocoa powder, and water and pour over batter.
5. Bake at 350°F/Gas Mark 4/180°C for 45 minutes. Serve hot or warm.

Makes 8 servings.
Per serving: 253 calories, 0 cholesterol, 1 g dietary fibre, 4 g fat, 234 mg sodium

Elegant Pears

This is especially good with coffee liqueur. Experiment with your favourite liqueurs.

2 large hard pears *or* 4 small
1¼ pints/700 ml water
6 tablespoons chocolate syrup or ice-cream topping

2 tablespoons liqueur of choice
small carton plain low-fat yoghurt or skimmed crème fraiche

1. Wash pears, cut in half and core. Bring water to boil. Add pear halves, reduce heat, and cover. Cook until pears are soft. Put yoghurt into ice-making compartment of fridge.
2. While pears are cooking, combine chocolate syrup and liqueur and heat in a small saucepan.
3. Drain pears and wipe off excess moisture. While still warm, top each pear half with 1 dessertspoon ice-cold yoghurt or crème fraiche. Pour approximately 2 tablespoons of chocolate syrup mixture over each. Serve immediately.

Makes 4 servings.
Per serving: 204 calories, 5 mg cholesterol, 3.5 g dietary fibre, 2 g fat, 58 mg sodium: approx. figures as British yoghurt and chocolate toppings differ from the American Hershey's syrup and ice milk used in the original recipe.

Lemon Meringue Pie

12 fl oz/330 ml measure plain or gingernut biscuit crumbs (about 6 oz/175 g)
2 dessertspoons honey
1 dessertspoon oil
10 oz/300 g sugar
3 dessertspoons cornflour
3 dessertspoons plain white flour

Dash of salt
12 fl oz/330 ml hot water
2 eggs, slightly beaten
½ teaspoon grated lemon peel
5 tablespoons lemon juice
3 egg whites
¼ teaspoon cream of tartar
¼ teaspoon vanilla essence
4 tablespoons castor sugar

1. Combine the biscuit crumbs, honey and oil. Mix well and press into a 9 inch/23 cm flan-tin. Bake for 10 minutes at 350°F/Gas Mark 4/180°C.
2. In a medium saucepan, combine the 10 oz/300 g sugar, the cornflour, flour and salt. Turn the heat to medium high and begin gradually adding the hot water, stirring constantly. Cook and stir until thickened and bubbly. Continue to cook 2 minutes longer.
3. Remove from heat. Stir a small amount of the hot mixture into the 2 beaten eggs, then add the mixture to the saucepan, return to heat, and cook 2 minutes more, stirring constantly.
4. Stir in lemon peel. Gradually add lemon juice, mixing well. Pour into prepared crust.
5. To make topping, beat egg whites with cream of tartar and vanilla essence until soft peaks form. Gradually add the 4 tablespoons of castor sugar, beating until glossy and mixture forms stiff peaks.

6. Spread on top of pie. Bake at 350°F/Gas Mark 4/180°C for about 12 minutes or until golden brown.

Makes 8 servings.
Per serving: 334 calories, 69 mg cholesterol, 2 g dietary fibre, 5.5 g fat, 176 mg sodium: approx figures as the fat and sugar content of biscuits varies. Check the packet for the lowest suitable kind.

*Poppy–seed Cake

4 tablespoons vegetable oil
5 oz/145 g sugar
2 eggs, separated
½ teaspoon vanilla essence
4 oz/110 g wholewheat flour
½ teaspoon salt

½ teaspoon soda bicarbonate
5 fl oz/150 ml plain low-fat
   yoghurt
5 tablespoons poppy seeds
Non-stick vegetable cooking oil

1. Blend the oil and sugar in a large bowl. Add the egg yolks one at a time, beating well. Add the vanilla essence.
2. In another bowl, sift together the flour, salt and soda bicarbonate. Alternatively fold the flour mixture and the yoghurt into the oil and and sugar mixture. Set aside.
3. Beat the egg whites until stiff. Fold into the batter. Fold in the poppy seeds.
4. Lightly oil an 8 inch/20 cm tube pan or bread-tin and dust lightly with whole-wheat flour. Pour the batter into the pan.
5. Bake at 350°F/Gas Mark 4/180°C for about 45–50 minutes, until top is nicely browned, and a toothpick inserted in the centre comes out clean.

Makes 20 servings.
Per serving: 131 calories, 34 mg cholesterol, 1 g dietary fibre, 7 g fat, 109 mg sodium

Pumpkin Cheesecake

12 fl oz/330 ml measure of biscuit
   crumbs (about 6 oz/175 g)
2 dessertspoons honey
1 dessertspoon oil
2 whole eggs
3 egg whites
8 oz/225 g of softened Neufchâtel
   or other soft cream cheese,
   low fat if possible

12 oz/350 g 'lite' ricotta cheese
4 fl oz/110 ml plain very low fat
   yoghurt
15 oz/425 g tin pumpkin, or
   1 lb/450 g raw
6 oz/175 g sugar
½ teaspoon vanilla essence
¼ teaspoon nutmeg
¼ teaspoon cinnamon

1. Combine the biscuit crumbs, honey and oil. Mix well and press into a lightly oiled 9-inch/23 cm flan-tin. Heat oven to 350°F/Gas Mark 4/180°C.
2. In a mixing bowl, beat together the eggs and egg whites until foamy. Add all other ingredients. Beat until smooth and creamy. (If using raw pumpkin, cook by baking in oven, covered, for about 1 hour at 325°F/Gas Mark 3/170°C. Remove pips and strings, then scrape pulp from shell.)
3. Pour into the crust and bake at 350° until slightly browned and firm in the centre, about 45 minutes.

Variations: Omit pumpkin, nutmeg and cinnamon. After baking, top with stoned cherries, or other fruit.

Makes 10 servings.
Per serving: 294 calories, 102 mg cholesterol, 2.5 g fibre, 12 g fat, 336 mg sodium: approx. figures as the fat content of both cheeses and biscuits will vary according to what is available to you.

CHAPTER SEVEN

THE T-FACTOR ACTIVITY PROGRAMME

I've heard it both ways. Successful people who have lost weight and are keeping it off say, 'It's the physical activity that's doing it. I'm not really dieting any more. My weight stays off as long as I'm active.' Unsuccessful people often say just the opposite: 'I started an activity programme. Three to five times a week, in fact. I didn't lose a pound. I even gained!'

Both are right. Exercise can be the key that makes weight management easy. However, under certain conditions, exercise can keep you fat. Exercise may even help you to gain weight – fat weight. I've talked with many people who have lost weight only to regain it despite religious attendance at their fitness and aerobic dancing classes.*

Before I explain how this can occur, I want to say, without qualification, that daily physical activity combined with the T-Factor Diet provides *an absolute guarantee that you will burn body fat and lose weight. In addition, continuing to apply T-Factor principles to your diet and activity programme is an absolute guarantee that you will not regain any weight.*

So, what are the conditions under which physical activity can

* We have had many people enter the Vanderbilt Weight Management Program who have regained weight after previous diets in spite of participation in fitness, calisthenics, and aerobic dance classes. However, no formal research of which I am aware clearly demonstrates how certain forms of exercise, in combination with a high-fat diet, promote weight gain. My discussion and the examples using myself in this chapter are based on other facts pertaining to exercise physiology and theory.

impede weight loss? How can I provide you with such a contrasting guarantee that you will lose weight and keep it off with the T-Factor Activity Programme?

Remember that the key to losing fat weight is to burn more fat in your fuel mixture each day than you take in through your diet. Under these conditions, the fat must be withdrawn from your fat cells. Obviously the converse is true: You will gain fat weight easily if you take in more fat than you are burning in your fuel mixture. The surplus fat in your diet ends up in your fat cells. The key is *fat in versus fat out*. The carbohydrate in your diet will play little part in gaining fat weight since so little of it, under normal circumstances, is turned to fat.

Can you see how someone who eats a high-fat diet – in fact, no higher than the typical Western diet – *may be replacing all the fat burned through physical activity because of that high-fat diet and end up never losing an ounce of fat weight?*

But the plot thickens. There is a rather complex relationship between diet and activity when it comes to reducing body fat.

Some physical activities do not use body fat as the major component of the fuel mixture that powers them. Other physical activities do. Unfortunately, many of the activity programmes that overweight people turn to in an effort to control their weight do not burn body fat as the major component of the fuel mixture.

PUT THE WRONG ACTIVITY PROGRAMME TOGETHER WITH THE TYPICAL WESTERN DIET AND YOU CAN PREVENT WEIGHT LOSS. INDEED, YOU MAY POSSIBLY GAIN WEIGHT!

FACTS ABOUT PHYSICAL ACTIVITY

Some activities burn fat as the major component in the fuel mixture. These activities are most helpful in controlling your weight. Some activities burn carbohydrate (glucose) as the major component in the fuel mixture. THESE ACTIVITIES CAN ALSO BE HELPFUL IN CONTROLLING BODY WEIGHT *PROVIDED* YOU ARE EATING ACCORDING TO T-FACTOR PRINCIPLES. However, if, after losing weight, you combine carbohydrate-burning exercise with a return to your previous high-fat eating habits, you can regain fat weight quite easily.

Here is how this works.

Start-stop activities at a moderate to vigorous intensity, sometimes referred to as anaerobic activities,* will burn in the vicinity of 60 to 70 per cent carbohydrate (in the form of glucose) in the fuel mixture, and 30 to 40 per cent fat. The more vigorous and taxing each spurt of activity, the more carbohydrate it requires. In fact, among top athletes, a 100-yard dash or a session of high-intensity interval training (alternating laps at top speed and recovery speed) can use 90 per cent or more of carbohydrate in the fuel mixture.

But most of us will never exercise at the very highest anaerobic intensity, so I will use the more conservative 60 to 70 per cent estimate for carbohydrate burned during our quick start-and-stop activities. Thus, most of us working about as hard as we can, sprinting in football, tennis or squash, and working out in most aerobic dance and calisthenic classes, will force our bodies to burn about 70 per cent carbohydrate during any given exercise period and only 30 per cent fat.

I'll show you how this kind of activity combined with an improper diet could lead to weight gain in a moment, but first let's contrast this with gentle jogging and brisk walking.

Steady-state activities which move your whole body through space or which require continuous movement of the largest muscles in your thighs and buttocks, sometimes called 'aerobic activities', *burn between 50 and 60 per cent fat in the fuel mixture and only about 40 to 50 per cent carbohydrate*. In steady-state aerobic activities that burn fat at this level, such as jogging and walking, your heart and breathing rates go up, level out, and stay there throughout the activity period. The activities are called aerobic because you burn fuel only as fast as you can supply oxygen for its combustion. The activity feels 'moderate' to you – you breathe harder, but you don't get 'out of breath'. You can do it for forty-five minutes to an hour and while you may get tired in that period of time, you do not become exhausted.

To summarize:

* Anaerobic activities happen so quickly that the energy which drives them is burned without the presence of oxygen. This is possible because your muscles store some fuel in a form that can be used even when the heart and circulating blood cannot supply enough fuel and oxygen to keep up with the demand. Start-stop activities of this kind, including calisthenics, aerobic dance, racket sports, weightlifting and other sports that require sprinting, are characterized by wide swings in your breathing and heart rates. Because these activities have burned fuel without the presence of oxygen, they put you into what is called an 'oxygen deficit'. That is, in order to catch up and restore energy to the emptied muscles, your heart must continue to beat rapidly and you must breathe more heavily for some time after you finish each burst of activity.

START-STOP ACTIVITIES ARE CARBOHYDRATE-BURNING ACTIVITIES. IN GENERAL, THEY WILL BURN BETWEEN 60 AND 70 PER CENT CARBOHYDRATE AND 30 TO 40 PER CENT FAT IN THE FUEL MIXTURE.

CONTINUOUS WHOLE-BODY MOVEMENTS ARE FAT-BURNING ACTIVITIES. THEY WILL BURN BETWEEN 50 AND 60 PER CENT FAT IN THE FUEL MIXTURE AND 40 TO 50 PER CENT CARBOHYDRATE.

For reference purposes I call the carbohydrate-fuelled activities 'carb burners' for short, and fat-fuelled activities are simply 'fat burners'.

To demonstrate how diet and activity interact and can either facilitate or interfere with fat loss, let's use tennis and brisk walking, with myself as an example.

In an hour of singles tennis I burn about 500 calories. That will be typical of a man weighing about 11 stone/70 kg (my present weight after adopting the T-Factor Diet) who plays at a strong competitive level and who spends his time chasing tennis balls rather than socializing or just picking the balls up after very short rallies. A woman weighing 2 stone/14 kg less than I do may burn only about 400 to 450 calories in the hour since it takes fewer calories to carry the lighter body around. Heavier people will burn more.

Assuming I play quite vigorously, about 70 per cent of the calories burned in an hour will come out of my glycogen stores and 30 per cent will come out of my fat stores. Thus, about 350 of the calories will be supplied by carbohydrate, and about 150 from fat.

When I walk briskly at 4 miles per hour (or 15 minutes per mile) I burn approximately 400 calories in an hour. This figure will be typical of a man weighing 11 stone/70 kg and, as before, a woman weighing 2 stone/14 kg less may burn 50 to 100 calories less in this period of time. Heavier people will burn more.

I am in pretty good shape and walking at 4 miles per hour elevates my heart rate only about 12 beats above my resting level. That is, it's a comfortable, steady-state aerobic activity. In an hour of walking, when compared with tennis, there will be a change in the ratio of fat to carbohydrate burned – I will burn up to about 60 per cent fat to 40 per cent carbohydrate. I will burn about 240 fat calories and 160 carbohydrate calories.

Summarizing again: In an hour of vigorous singles tennis I will burn about 350 calories in carbohydrate and 150 calories in fat; in an hour of walking I will burn 160 calories in carbohydrate and 240 calories in fat.

Now, it is important to remember, first of all, that the depletion of carbohydrate in my muscles and liver stores is a stronger factor in the arousal of appetite than is the loss of fat from my fat cells.* I am likely to be somewhat hungrier after tennis than after walking. But much more important in determining whether I gain or lose fat is whether I am eating a high-fat diet or following the T-Factor Diet.

If I eat a high-fat diet such as is consumed by the majority of overweight people in the Western world, which contains about 40 per cent of calories from fat and 45 percent from carbohydrate, by the time I have replaced the 350 carbohydrate calories I will also have eaten $^8/_9$ths as much fat, or roughly about 310 fat calories ($^{40}/_{45}$ = $^8/_9$). *That's 160 more fat calories than I burned during the exercise.*

Unless I find a way to burn more fat than carbohydrate during the rest of the day, I am going to gain weight.

If your weight has been stable on an exercise programme that emphasizes carbohydrate-burning activity, it means that you do burn more fat than carbohydrate during the rest of the day. This compensation is possible because just sitting still or sleeping, while not burning many calories at all, still burns a bit more fat than carbohydrate. You do tend to sit and sleep for longer than you dance or stretch.

But if you have gained weight after losing it on a calorie-reduced diet and you expected your calisthenics, dance class, or tennis match to prevent it, now you know why your exercise programme didn't work.

Now let's take a look at what happens when brisk walking is combined with the T-Factor Diet. I'll use myself again as an example when I first adopted the T-Factor Diet, when walking was my only exercise activity.

When I limited fat intake to about 60 grams a day, I tended to eat about 65 per cent of calories from carbohydrates, 15 per cent from protein, and about 20 per cent from fat. In other words, I was taking in about 3 calories of carbohydrate for every calorie of fat. By the time I'd replaced the 160 calories of carbohydrate that I used in walking for an hour, I had eaten only 50 to 60 calories in fat. This meant that in order to satisfy the need to refill my glycogen stores, I ended up eating only about 220 calories in all (160 to replace the carbohydrate plus about 60 in fat), which, theoretically, should have resulted in a loss of about 180 calories from my fat stores in that hour of activity (240 fat calories burned during the hour's walk, with 60 replaced). I am sure this emphasis on fat-burning activity during my injury period played a role in losing those 7 pounds (3 kg), as I described in Chapter Four.

The T-Factor formula is also protecting me from weight gain now that I have resumed playing tennis. Since I am adhering to the

---

* The role of glycogen depletion in the arousal of appetite is discussed in Chapter Ten.

same 3 to 1 ratio of carbohydrate to fat in my diet, by the time I have replaced the 350 carbohydrate calories burned in an hour of tennis, I do not consume more fat than the 150 or so fat calories that burned in the fuel mixture during the game. Thus I do not regain any weight.

Can you also see how fat burners make it so much easier to take off body fat and keep it off when they are combined with the T-Factor Diet? When you focus primarily on maximum fat-burning activities in your exercise programme, and combine this with a low-fat, high-carbohydrate diet, you keep your glycogen stores at maximum, your appetite satisfied and your body fat at its healthiest minimum.

THE IDEAL FAT-BURNING ACTIVITY PROGRAMME

The fitter you are, the more fat you burn!

Take any aerobic activity: walking, jogging, bicycling, swimming, rowing, cross-country skiing or any other continuous whole-body movement. If you are out of shape, brisk movement will require considerable effort. You will burn carbohydrate as the principal component in your fuel mixture when you first begin to engage in any of these activities. However, as you increase in fitness, *all these activities become fat burners*.

How do you develop the ideal fat-burning activity programme and increase fitness?

From a physiological standpoint, the ideal programme consists in part of a combination of exercises that vary in intensity. This is necessary because, in order to build endurance so that higher levels of exertion begin to feel more and more moderate, you have to exert yourself occasionally.

Here is an example of how walking was transformed from a carb to fat burner, and how it was done by a group of overweight women in the Vanderbilt Weight Management Program. The research subjects were in their thirties and forties and approximately 4½ stone (27 kg) overweight on the average. On the first test walk at 3 miles per hour (20 minutes per mile), their heart rates averaged 138 beats per minute (BPM) and most of the women were tired and needed to stop after only 20 minutes. Walking at this level of exertion was, for them, a carbohydrate-burning activity.

Over the next 12 weeks the women walked 6 days a week, with two objectives: increase time to 45 minutes, then increase speed. In order to increase speed, as their condition improved, they began to intersperse periods of brisk walking at a 4-mph pace (15 minutes per mile). By the end of the 12 weeks, all the women were able to walk for 45 minutes at 3 mph without stopping, and many could maintain a 4-mph pace for a good part of the time.

We then did a second test at the 3-mph pace. Their heart rates at this pace had decreased to 112 beats per minute. Walking at 3 mph had become a fat-burning activity, and I estimate that the percentage of fat burned while walking at this pace increased from 30 to at least 50 per cent.

THUS, AS PHYSICAL CONDITION IMPROVES, THE FAT-BURNING POTENTIAL OF SIMILAR CONTINUOUS WHOLE-BODY MOVEMENT IMPROVES.

In addition, because the women had been able to increase total walking each day from approximately 1 mile to 3 miles, on average, the total number of fat calories burned in activity increased significantly: from about 30 (of the total 100 burned in about 20 minutes of walking at the start of the programme) to about 150 (of the total 300 burned in the 45 to 60 minutes at the end of 12 weeks).

FAT BURNING WAS THUS ABOUT FIVE TIMES HIGHER THAN AT THE START OF THE WALKING PRO-GRAMME. This is why physical activity of the fat-burning type is so important to weight loss and maintenance. IN ADDITION, BECAUSE TOTAL ACTIVITY WAS GREATER, THEY WERE ABLE TO BURN EVEN MORE CARBOHYDRATE THAN AT THE START OF THE PROGRAMME. With daily physical activity you can truly eat more, including more carbo-hydrate, and still draw more and more body fat from storage and end up weighing less.

Although we know that you will burn more fat calories relative to carbohydrate calories as your condition improves and your heart rate goes down in any physical activity at a given intensity, as it did in the women in my example, it is not possible to give you a precise estimate of the fat-burning to carbohydrate-burning ratio of physi-cal activities by heart rate. It is an entirely individual matter that can only be determined in the laboratory. By that I mean that the same heart rate in two different individuals can have an entirely different implication with respect to both total calories burned in any unit of time and the ratio of fat to glucose burned in the fuel mixture.

But you can be sure of this as you become more active: *In any steady-state activity, as your cardiovascular condition improves, any decrease in heart rate for a given intensity of exercise means more fat burned.*

You can increase your cardiovascular endurance by exercising periodically in what is called the 'training range'.

THE TRAINING HEART RATE

You can get a rough idea of both your physical condition and your fat-burning ratio from a consideration of what is called the 'training heart rate'.

Although some kind of moderate to brisk physical activity almost every day for 45 minutes to an hour is extremely helpful if not essential to weight management, if you wish to improve cardiovascular fitness to a greater extent and achieve a high level of fat-burning potential in your more moderate physical activity, you must occasionally exercise at a more intense level.

You can achieve significant cardiovascular benefits by getting your heart rate into the 'training range' about four times a week for about 20 to 30 minutes each time. That's all it takes. Any whole-body movement, or use of the major muscles in your buttocks and thighs, that you can perform continuously for that period of time is about as good as any other: walking, bicycling, swimming, rowing (including leg movement) or gentle jogging if you are already at desirable weight. When you exercise in the training range, you bring your heart to a level of exertion that increases its capacity to pump blood with each beat while at the same time increasing the ability of your circulatory system to handle the increased blood flow. In addition, the oxygen-carrying capacity of the blood is increased as well as the ability of your muscles to extract that oxygen and use it to power physical movement. All this means that physical activity at any given level of intensity begins to feel easier and easier.

For example, at very high levels of fitness, runners experience little or no elevation in heart rate when going from sitting to walking. In my own case, my heart rate goes from about 54 beats per minute while sitting to 60 when walking at 3 miles per hour and to about 66 at 4 miles per hour. The average sedentary person who embarks on a walking fitness programme will notice, at around 12 weeks, about a 20 per cent reduction in cardiovascular effort while walking at any given speed (just like the women in my example above). Frequently, but not always, there is a reduction in resting heart rate as well.

There is a simple rule of thumb that you can use to bring your heart into its training range.

Subtract your age from 220.

(On average, that will be about the fastest your heart can beat during an all-out sprint. Speed decreases with age.)

Multiply that figure by 0.60 (which is 60 per cent).

The figure you obtain is the low end of the training range.

Multiply the same figure (220 minus your age) by 0.85 (which is 85 per cent).

That is the high end of your training range.

If you exercise within this range for 20 to 30 minutes, four times a week, you will soon begin to experience an improvement in cardio-vascular fitness.

To measure your improvement, take your pulse at certain levels of exertion – for example, while walking at 3 and at 4 miles per hour. Over time you will find that your heart rate decreases while performing the same intensity of exercise.

Table 7.1 presents the training levels for age groups by five-year increments in age.

TABLE 7.1
MAXIMUM HEART RATES AND TRAINING RANGES

Age	Maximum Heart Rate (beats per minute)	60% Level (beats per minute)	85% Level (beats per minute)
20	200	120	170
25	195	117	166
30	190	114	162
35	185	111	157
40	180	108	153
45	175	105	149
50	170	102	145
55	165	99	140
60	160	96	136
65	155	93	132
70	150	90	128

STARTING OUT

When you first begin a training programme, stick to the low end of the training range, and do not exceed the upper level of your training range. To achieve very high levels of fitness, however, you do have to exercise at the high end of the training range for 20 to 30 minutes four times a week. Only people in excellent condition should do this, and if you are overweight and out of condition you should definitely check with your doctor if you intend to exercise strenuously. It can be dangerous for people with cardiovascular disease and overweight people may be somewhat more likely to have undiagnosed cardiovascular disease than thin people.

REMEMBER THE FIRST RULE OF FITNESS: NEVER HURT YOURSELF!

While world-class athletes must tax themselves to reach maximum levels of skill and fitness, good health does not demand it. In fact, I don't know of any world-class athlete who has not at one time or another had an injury that interfered with training for at least a brief period of time. That's the price they must pay to win championships. Unfortunately, their injuries may haunt them for the rest of their lives and actually be detrimental to their health in the long run. You and I don't need to go to such extremes.

MAKING PROGRESS

As your condition improves, test yourself at somewhat higher levels of exertion. Listen to your body. Pain is a signal to slow down. A feeling of greater effort, without pain, is not. However, a bit of *strain*, not pain, is required to reach higher levels of fitness. When you get comfortable exercising at the 60 per cent level in the training range, experiment with reaching up to the 70 or 75 per cent level. That's quite high enough. Do not continue in the face of pain. In the end, you can hurt yourself and not be able to exercise at all for a period of time. That can be demoralizing and depressing.

Whatever activity you choose, and I will recommend walking at first, pay special attention to muscular aches and pains. Musculoskeletal injury is the most likely kind of injury at the start of an exercise programme. There is also an increased likelihood of injury any time you make a sudden increase in intensity or duration. Moderation and gradual progress should be your guide words.

WHY WALK FOR HEALTH AND SLIMNESS?

Any continuous whole-body movement is about as good as any other for burning body fat and for combining with the T-Factor Diet for permanent weight management.

Walking is easiest and most convenient for most people. Walking burns more calories with less perceived effort than other activities. That's because most of us do at least a little walking every day and that gives us a base to build on. At 3 mph we burn about 100 total calories every 20 minutes. At 4 mph we burn about 100 total calories every 15 minutes.

If walking is impossible for you, then bicycling or rowing, in which you move your legs as well as your arms, is excellent. However, it requires more perceived effort to burn the same number of calories on a bicycle or on a rowing machine until you become accustomed to those means of exercise. Ski machines can also be good, but don't believe the exaggerated claims for calorie burning that some manufacturers make. No one but highly trained athletes can approach even 1,000 calories an hour of energy expenditure, much less 600 in 200 minutes.

And, by the way, fitness for exercise is quite specific to each exercise. As a jogger, I hardly notice my heart rate after an hour at a pace of a mile in 10 minutes (6 mph), but at the same level of oxygen consumption on a bicycle I feel considerable strain in my legs after only 20 minutes. That's because I don't use the leg or buttock muscles in the same way for jogging as I do on a bicycle. And when it comes to swimming freestyle one length of an Olympic-sized pool I'm out of breath. I occasionally ride a bicycle, but I never swim even though swimming is an excellent exercise. I just don't care for it. However, despite the claims of some experts that swimming won't work for weight loss and might even lead to an increase in body-fat storage, *swimming can be an excellent aid to weight management and overall health and fitness*. I will dispel some myths about swimming below.

If you choose walking as your T-Factor activity, use the principle of gradualness and start by walking about 15 minutes at a time, at whatever pace feels good to you. *Increase time before you increase your speed*.

Work up to 45 minutes or an hour over a one- or two-month period. For both physiological and psychological reasons (the latter are discussed in Chapter Eight), I don't think you can ever fall in love with physical activity of any kind unless you learn to do it well and do it or some other alternating activity for at least 45 minutes to an hour *on an almost daily basis. And the activity or activities must end up feeling easy to you.*

As you recall, however, for training purposes, you must occasionally exert yourself. The rules call for you to kick yourself up to a brisk pace for 20 minutes or so, four times a week. As your condition improves, this will result in a feeling of tremendous exhilaration, not exhausation. For training purposes, check your heart rate occasionally to see that during the periods in which you increase speed you are actually obtaining training benefits. However, walking is primarily a time to escape the regimentation you may be obliged to apply to the rest of your daily activities. I think you should feel free to bend the rules because, in my experience, people accomplish more by using a whimsical training approach and a 'feeling good' principle rather than any mathematical formula or mechanical method. Listen to your body and whenever it says go faster, GO. And when it says slow down, SLOW DOWN.

As I said before, the fitter you get, the more fat you burn in any given aerobic activity. Even without fussing over your heart rate, you can tell that the ratio of fat to carbohydrate that is being burned is increasing when, at any given intensity, the feeling of effort decreases.

And now another important point:

THE LONGER YOU GO THE MORE FAT YOU BURN.

When you first start out in any activity, including walking and other aerobic activities, a major part of the fuel mix is drawn from your glycogen pool. As you continue moving in the steady state, your body switches tanks, as it were, and begins to draw from its fat stores. The fitter you are, the sooner the switch takes place; and the longer you go, the more fat relative to glycogen you will use. This is one reason why walking for an hour is better than walking for twelve different 5-minute segments during the day. BUT IF BRIEF WALKS ARE ALL YOU CAN MANAGE MOST OF THE TIME, DO THEM. THEN, TRY TO GET A FEW LONGER WALKS IN DURING THE WEEK SO THAT YOUR FITNESS WILL IMPROVE. THIS WILL MAXIMIZE FAT BURNING EVEN IN YOUR SHORTER WALKS.

Once again let me emphasize the importance of the T-Factor Diet in any case where physical activity cannot be pursued for at least 45 minutes at a stretch, or where carb burners form a major part of your exercise programme.

I am sure that you are interested in having a list of activities that indicates the ratio of fat to carbohydrate that tends to be burned in the fuel mixture. You will find this in Table 7.2, where I list approximate calories burned per 15 minutes according to standard tables and indicate which activities are fat burners. Outside the laboratory, however, it is impossible to determine the exact ratio of

TABLE 7.2

APPROXIMATE ENERGY COSTS IN EACH 15 MINUTES OF VARIOUS ACTIVITIES*

Activity	Calories per 15 minutes
Aerobic dancing	105
Badminton	99
*Ballroom dancing, continuous	53
Basketball	141
*Canoeing (recreational)	45
*Climbing hills (steady pace)	123
*Cooking	47
*Cycling	
5.5 mph, level ground	66
9.4 mph, level ground	102
Football	135

TABLE 7.2 *cont.*

Activity	Calories per 15 minutes
*Gardening (raking)	56
*Golf (walking – no cart)	87
Gymnastics	88
*Horseback riding	
walking	42
trotting (posting)	113
*Housework (steady movement)	63
Judo	199
*Piano playing	41
*Rowing (machine, fast pace)	105
*Running	
11 min. 30 sec. per mile	138
10 min. per mile	174
9 min. per mile	197
8 min. per mile	213
7 min. per mile	234
6 min. per mile	260
Skiing	
*cross-country, walking pace	146
downhill	101
Squash	216
*Swimming	
freestyle, moderate pace	143
sidestroke	125
Table tennis	69
Tennis	111
*Typing (electric typewriter)	27
Volleyball	51
*Walking	
3 mph, level ground	66
4 mph, level ground	99
downstairs, steady pace	50
upstairs, slow steady pace	151

* Energy costs are calculated for people weighing 14 stone 10 pounds (68 kg). For each 10 pounds (4.5 kg) more or less, add or subtract 7 per cent, respectively. Activities marked with an asterisk (*) are fat burners – between 50 and 60 per cent of the calories listed will be withdrawn from your fat cells. About 30 per cent of the calories listed for unmarked items are fuelled by fat.

fat to carbohydrate that is being burned in any given case because there are such large individual differences, some of which, as you now know, are a function of fitness level. The figures given in the footnote to the table assume a level of fitness that you will reach if you customarily perfom that particular activity.

AN INCREASE IN EXERCISE TIME OR INTENSITY CAN LEAD TO A BRIEF GAIN OF A FEW POUNDS

If at any time you get turned on and suddenly increase your exercise time or intensity a significant amount, say, by 50 per cent, you may gain a couple of pounds overnight. This will be gone in a matter of one to two days. It occurs because a sudden increase in exercise – increasing your walking from 3 to 4½ miles at the weekend, for example – will cause your exercised muscles to take in an extra load of glycogen from subsequent meals. Since glycogen is stored with 3 to 4 parts water, it means a considerable weight gain. I gained 2 pounds (1 kg) overnight when I took my first 6-mile run after being accustomed to only 2 or 3 miles per session.

Similarly, if you develop any aches or pains, accompanied by any inflammation of the muscles or joints, it means a gain in water weight since the inflamed area will retain some water.

WHAT ABOUT TIME OF DAY?

Any time that's best for you, in terms of convenience and good feelings, is always the best time to exercise.

But there is evidence that exercise before meals burns the most body fat. That's because the body tends to adjust its fuel mixture to the diet and, immediately after a typical high-carbohydrate T-Factor meal, will tend to burn additional carbohydrate. Before meals, your glycogen stores are relatively low, and to conserve glycogen, your body tends to increase its use of fat as fuel.

The combination of walking before meals, which will maximize fat in the fuel mix, and sticking to the T-Factor Diet, which replaces glycogen without replacing the burned fat, will lead to the quickest and greatest permanent fat loss.

Because you are at your lowest ebb in glycogen storage before breakfast, walking before breakfast may lead to the greatest use of fat as fuel. This will be especially true after a cup of coffee or other caffeinated beverage. Caffeine increases the flow of fatty acids from your fat cells. However, if drinking coffee or walking on a completely empty stomach makes you uncomfortable, try eating a slice of toast or a few crispbreads first. This is what I do before my morning walk or jog. I feel much better with a little something more than coffee inside.

EXERCISE AND APPETITE

Depending on a number of factors, exercise can either decrease or increase appetite.

In sedentary people who are out-eating their energy needs and gaining weight, exercise may help reduce non-hunger-related overeating. Exercise, by raising body temperature, decreasing the flow of saliva, and diverting blood from the internal organs to the muscles, decreases appetite in the short term. Then, when appetite returns after exercise, it seems to be better attuned to the amount of energy you are expending each day than it is in the sedentary person. In other words, people who exercise tend to eat in a way that does not lead to an increase in weight. It's as though Mother Nature, in ways that we are unaware of, keeps our bodies adapted to the physical demands we make on them. The active person needs a thinner body in order to be efficient in activity, so appetite becomes regulated to keep you thin. This mysterious adaptive mechanism goes awry in the sedentary person.

But certain forms of exercise, under certain conditions, can also increase appetite beyond its accustomed level. You recall that appetite is, to a large extent, regulated by our glycogen stores. With a steady, ongoing exercise programme to which we have become accustomed, glycogen stores fluctuate within the accustomed range together with our appetites, and all is in balance. But we can exceed the usual range and become really hungry when we make a drastic change in the nature of our activity.

This was brought home to me the very first time I did a complete strength-training workout under the guidance of an instructor at the YMCA. He was demonstrating the equipment in the weight room, so that I would know what to do on future visits, and I did several sets of exercises covering both the lower and upper body. I did all exercises to virtual exhaustion for all the muscle groups. (Normally you would do upper body on one day, lower body on another.)

I went to my office at the university after the workout, and about an hour or so later I became ravenous. I have rarely had such an appetite in my life. It was a completely different sensation compared with other times when I have been hungry after going a long time between meals. It reduced me to near criminal activity: I went sneaking around the psychology department, looking for food in my colleagues' offices and in the secretaries' offices. I think the near complete depletion of my muscle glycogen stores was responsible for this. In addition, there may have been an increased need for some protein for muscle repairs, since this was the first time I had ever lifted weights.

Fortunately, one of the secretaries had a packet of peanut butter crackers(!), which she gave to me, and my appetite was satisfied until lunch. But once again, as with the sudden increase in running mileage, my glycogen stores were replenished above baseline and I ended up a couple of pounds heavier the next day.

Will strength training interfere with weight loss and fat loss on the T-Factor Diet?

Power lifting – that is, heavy weight lifting with quick explosive movements to exhaustion for each muscle group – burns primarily carbohydrate in the fuel mixture. If you want to lose weight and body fat, and you include weight lifting in your regimen, YOU MUST BE SURE THAT YOU FOLLOW THE T-FACTOR DIET in order to replenish carbohydrate without an overconsumption of fat, since weight lifting is not a fat-burning activity. I do, however, encourage you to follow my moderate endurance strength-training programme (Appendix B) becuase it will tone you up and you will look and feel better for doing it. Light endurance training, rather than power lifting, will not affect fat loss or weight loss adversely.

Should you walk with weights in your hands or use some artificial 'power' motion? I would approach both of these options cautiously. Carrying light weights (1 lb/450 g) can help improve cardiovascular condition more rapidly and build a little more muscular endurance, but I have known people to sustain joint injuries and lower back pain by adding weights while they walked. Race walking, however, has been a life saver for many joggers who have injured themselves running, so if you learn the motion correctly, you probably won't injure yourself race walking. Simply swinging your arms any old way that feels good to you while walking can significantly increase the intensity of your workout and build endurance. Test out all changes in your changes in your natural walking style gingerly, and let your experience be your guide.

THE SWIMMING CONTROVERSY

Noted experts have claimed that you can't lose body fat if you take up swimming as the main component of your exercise programe. This is simply not true.

The reason some experts claim that swimming is not a good exercise for weight control is that the temperature of the pool, being perhaps 20 or more degrees cooler than your body, encourages the body to retain the layer of surface fat that lies just under your skin. In thin people who may have little to begin with, swimming may help add a bit of surface fat. This occurs to help prevent heat loss as your body struggles to maintain its internal temperature at around 98.4°F/37°C.

However, swimming, when it becomes as easy as walking or jogging for you, is actually a fat-burning exercise, and the struggle to maintain internal temperature is also fuelled by fat to a large extent. In combination with the T-Factor Diet, you are assured of burning more fat in your fuel mixture than you are eating if you make swimming your favourite exercise. But you *will* tend to retain a bit more surface body fat than if you walk, jog or ride a bicycle.

Although I have never learned to be comfortable in the water, I have talked to people for whom swimming is as easy and automatic as walking. They can become completely entranced as they glide back and forth in the pool. It's as restful and refreshing as meditation for them. If you have difficulty coordinating your breathing with your strokes and this prevents you from becoming relaxed and enjoying a swim, you may find that learning to use a snorkel will put you completely at ease.

HOW TO DETERMINE THE EQUIVALENCE OF DIFFERENT EXERCISES

I am often asked how a person can determine the equivalence, in terms of calories or fat burned, when they perform different exercises. The best way to do this is to use your pulse rate as your guide. It's done in this way:

Go for a walk at 3 miles per hour (1 mile in 20 minutes) and, after about 5 minutes, measure your pulse rate. Walking at 3 mph burns about three times the calories of sitting still. Assuming a 50/50 ratio of fat to carbohydrate in your fuel mixture, it burns three times the fat as well as three times the carbohydrate as sitting still. Whenever you reach this pulse rate in any other activity in which you are reasonably comfortable, you will be burning about the same number of calories as you do while walking at 3 mph, and half those calories are coming out of your fat cells.

If you are capable of it, walk for 5 minutes at 4 mph (1 mile in 15 minutes) and take your pulse rate. Walking at 4 mph burns almost five times the calories of sitting still, and, assuming that you are in good condition, we can again assume about 50/50 mixture of fat to carbohydrate in your fuel mixture.* Whenever you reach this pulse rate in any other activity in which you are reasonably comfortable, you will be burning about the same number of calories as you do while walking at 4 mph, and about half of these are supplied by fat. Of course the fitter you get, the more fat you burn relative to carbohydrate.

THE COMPLETE FITNESS PROGRAMME

I have focused my discussion of physical activity on its role in regulating body fat because that is where our main interest lies. But staying fit and healthy also requires that we maintain our flexibility and muscular strength.

The masters of Yoga say, 'You are as old as your spine.' That's because, as we age, our spines, as well as other joints, lose flexibility. With loss of flexibility comes an increased likelihood of injury, together with the chronic aches and pains associated with stiffness. To a great extent, however, we can maintain flexibility and agility with appropriate stretching and toning exercises, and in this way we preserve biological if not chronological youth.

While many of us neglect to include a good stretching routine in our fitness programmes, even more fail to do anything to maintain muscular strength. The requirements of life today, for most of us, do not include much lifting or pushing of heavy objects. In fact, the heaviest thing most of us every carry after our children are grown up is the weekly bag of groceries. This means that we do not build and maintain a level of strength that can protect us from injury

---

* A person who is in good condition will be at the low end of, or even below, the training range in heart rate at this speed of walking. If, however, you reach your maximum heart rate, or the top end of your training range, you are burning primarily carbohydrate in your mixture. Many of the participants in aerobic dance classes are actually working out at maximum heart rates and burning as much as 90 per cent carbohydrate in their fuel mixtures. Only the instructor in the class is usually in good enough condition to be burning a high-fat fuel mixture.

whenever we find it necessary to exert physical force – even moving a chair, much less a heavier piece of furniture.

You can never experience a fraction of the energy, agility and vitality you are capable of unless you incorporate a modest level of stretching exercise and strength training into your regimen. In Appendix B I include a training routine that combines flexibility and modest strength-training exercises.

After you get a sense of what you need to do to maintain flexibility and strength, you can be creative and invent ways to do exercise of this nature and keep it interesting. Here's how I manage it.

A few stretches are essential to keep my back, hips, and leg joints flexible. They must be first in my morning ritual, or I run the danger of becoming too stiff or even injuring myself when I play tennis. Then, two or three times a week, when I am either walking or jogging in the woods near my home, I carry a tree branch that weighs about 6 pounds (2½ kg) and invent various exercises to do with it as I move along. At certain points on some routes, I've left large branches weighing 2 stone (11 kg) or so for more serious weight lifting. At other points I come across picnic tables, which I use to do additional stretches. These exercises have now become part of my routine along these trials and it is hard for me to pass by the appointed spots without doing them.

You now have the facts about exercise that can help you maximize your ability to burn fat, lose weight, and keep it off. I hope these facts and other hints for incorporating exercise in your life, will motivate you to begin an effective and enjoyable exercise programme. *I know that the reward from a correct programme is well worth the investment of time, cost of appropriate clothing and equipment, and physical effort.*

My problem lies in motivating you. I am well aware that facts about its health benefits are often not enough to sustain the will to exercise. Unfortunately, most people who begin an exercise programme in any given year do not continue it the next. If this has been your experience, I think the key to success for you, as for me, may lie in the psychological aspects of exercise. This is the subject of the next chapter.

CHAPTER EIGHT

PSYCHOLOGICAL ASPECTS OF EXERCISE AND FITNESS

Have you ever been so fat and out of shape that you had difficulty getting up out of a chair? It doesn't do much for your self-esteem.

Twenty-six years ago I was a fat man. I weighed over 16 stone (104 kg), which is about 5 stone (34 kg) more than I weigh today. I was so out of shape that I got out of breath walking a hundred yards or so and up one flight of stairs to the library close to my office of Vanderbilt. I so much hated to get out of my chair that I saved my library work for Friday afternoons in order to make only one trip per week. I was hypertensive and ended up with a minor coronary at the age of thirty-five.

I wish I could take the feeling I have inside me today and put it inside all the fat people in this world who hate exercise. If I could, you would never be fat again!

It's twenty-six years later, and jogs of 5 or 10 miles in the woods are easier today than that hated short walk to the library back in 1963. How did this happen?

There is no question that in many respects I went through a personality transformation. In a matter of two years I changed from someone who had never engaged in any physical activity at any period of his life to an amateur tennis player who began to enter and even win tournaments. True enough, I began to exercise for health reasons, but, like the great majority of people who begin an activity programme for the sake of their health, I would have given up if something much more motivating hadn't occurred as a result of becoming a tennis player and playing every day.

I don't think that any amount of lecturing on the physical benefits of exercise, either for weight control or for cardiovascular

179

health, will ever motivate the majority of sedentary people to become consistently active individuals. THE KEY IS PSYCHOLOGICAL AND EMOTIONAL.

In spite of all the important information I've given you in the previous chapter on the fat-burning benefits of exercise, I don't think you will succeed in becoming an active person who finds the joy in physical activity that I experience unless you find some activity that contributes to your self-concept and builds up your self-esteem. There is no question about it: Being a good tennis player and having the strength and endurance to jog easily for miles are, for me, an ego trip. What a contrast with my self-concept as a fat kid, 3½ stone (23 kg) overweight at the age of twelve, so ashamed of my looks that I wouldn't wear shorts. Indeed, so embarrassed with the look of my legs at the age of thirty-five that it took a whole year on the tennis courts before I discarded long trousers and bought my first pair of tennis shorts.

I do not exercise because it keeps me thin. I do not exercise because it may help prevent another heart attack (knock on wood, it must be helping so far). I run and play because running and playing contribute as much to the way I think about myself and describe myself as do being a college professor, health professional and writer or, for that matter, a husband and father.

Words can't communicate my experience, and the experience I wish you may have. There is an old Oriental proverb which states that there are some things that you can know only by doing. This is one of them.

Here is what you must do.

1. First you have to believe me. You must believe it's possible. Somewhere inside you, you must find the fantasy about yourself that can be fulfilled by developing the body and physical skills that you are about to cultivate.

2. You must do something physical every day. Only DOING can transform your BEING. The key word here is DISCIPLINE. But I don't intend any sense of harsh control or punishment when I use that word. I mean discipline in the sense of your becoming committed to a course of self-directed training that will mould and perfect your mental and physical character. I repeat: Your training sessions must happen every day.

3. You will never experience the 'flow', that is, the transformation of your physical state from sluggish to vital, from tense to relaxed, from tired to refreshed, unless just about every day you move about briskly for at least 45 minutes, and preferably for an hour at a time.

4. You must decide on some standard of performance. It has to

be one that is yours alone, no one else's. You must choose some standard that you are certain to reach, so that each day your chosen activity takes place as a ritual that can be completed. The standard can involve time, distance or speed, but it must be reachable and provide a sense of accomplishment.

5. If you choose some activity that is performed alone, it should not require much skill. Fortunately, the fat burners do not require Olympic-level athletic ability.

6. If you choose to engage in competitive activities, you must become as good as time and resources allow. For example, if you ever wanted to be a tennis player, it means lessons and practice. If you engage in the sport in the manner I suggest, you are out to become as good as you can be, which is quite different from going out to win every match. The joy must be found in the game itself, not the outcome.

7. It will take you at least a year, possibly even two years, to experience fully what I'm talking about. You must therefore be prepared to endure a kind of probationary status for this period of time. It will help from a psychological standpoint if you think of yourself as a novitiate. You will need to learn how to get through the change of seasons and the time changes each year. Depending on your choice of activity and the climate where you live, you may need to learn how to deal with the heat and the cold, the rain and the snow, the dogs along your route and the other vocational and social demands in your life. One day, you will realize that you are no longer a novitiate, but an 'initiate'; you will have become the person you set out to be.

8. If you choose physical activities that are social in nature, you must choose partners who are as enthusiastic as yourself. Drop those who disappoint you by not keeping appointments or who try to involve you in supporting their excuses for inactivity. You want partners for whom it is never too hot or too cold to be active!

9. Finally, if you choose some solo activity like walking, jogging or swimming (and I hope you do, at least as part of your total programme), you may have to experiment a bit to find an approach to this activity that leads to the kind of personal growth I'm speaking of. If you normally spend a great deal of time alone, then walking with friends can become an interesting social activity. There are walking groups in many cities, and you can always ask your neighbours if they would like to become walking companions. If you normally work with other people, or are under tension when you work, then walking alone is going to provide you with the greatest benefits. When I have been successful in persuading people to complete their probationary status, and get through a

year or two of walking or jogging, they almost always tell me that it has been a period of discovery. While they might have been bored at first, they discovered that walking alone provided them with an opportunity to consult themselves. They found an opportunity to consider thoughts, emotions, plans, hopes and dreams that could never have occurred otherwise. They got to know themselves, but best of all, they grew to like themselves a great deal better than before.

That's the final component. Simply put, you will know what I mean about self-esteem when you can say to yourself, 'The reason I walk [jog, play tennis, dance] is that I feel a better person for having done it.'

CHAPTER NINE

THE T-FACTOR PROGRAMME FOR CHILDREN AND ADOLESCENTS*

If you were ever fat as a child, as I was, you know at first hand the tremendous psychological and social burdens of childhood obesity. As a fat child, you're certain it's your fault that you're fat and that it reflects some sort of moral failure. You feel unattractive, of course, and you sense that everyone around you thinks you are, too.† Unless you have some special talent, you expect to be chosen last whenever teams are chosen during or after school.

Can you remember what it was like trying to buy clothes? In my home town there was only one shop back in the 1940s that had 'stouts' for fat kids like me, 3½ stone (23 kg) overweight at the age of twelve. I couldn't bear to look in the mirror after the assistant and my mother had forced me to try something on. I knew I looked fat and ugly no matter what they said. The damn suits were not slimming! My rear end was just as big as it was before I tried the trousers on.

Can you remember your first diet? If you were never fat as a child, and are trying to deal with one of your children who has a weight problem, you have no idea what it feels like to be 'put on a diet' as a kid when everyone else is free to eat as they please. You still live in a fat-eating environment. Nothing at school or after

---

* Much of the material for this chapter, including many of the tips for helping children either lose weight or maintain desirable weight, was furnished by Ms Jamie Pope-Cordle, MS, RD, director of nutrition, Vanderbilt Weight Management Program.

† Research shows that children as young as six years of age consider obese children to be less attractive than children with severe physical handicaps.

changes. Your friends all eat just as they ate before, in the school cafeteria and in the fast-food restaurants where the typical meal or snack contains from 40 to 55 per cent of its calories in fat. And, most likely, nothing at home changes, either, except for more arguments about food and dieting. You are still surrounded from the moment you wake up in the morning until the moment you go to sleep by all the fatty foods that tempt you. Your mother still cooks exactly as she did before and, suddenly, because you must be 'on a diet', you are supposed to have more willpower than a saint – certainly more than anyone else in your family.

Unless you have been there, I don't think you can appreciate that for most overweight children the situation is really quite desperate and sad. Perhaps you might have answered as the overweight child of one of the participants in the Vanderbilt Weight Management Program did when his school counsellor asked him what he wished for more than anything else in the world. Yes, perhaps you guessed – 'To be thin.'

Well, he's had his wish granted because his mother took home everything she had learned when she lost weight in the T-Factor programme and decided to make it a family affair. In a moment I'll give you the advice that worked for this family because it can work for you, too. First some basics.

WE DO NOT BELIEVE IN PUTTING CHILDREN AND ADOLESCENTS ON DIETS.

A vast number of children, perhaps a majority, come to believe that weight control is a matter of going on and off diets. I see it in many of the young men and women in my classes at Vanderbilt who are not overweight, as well as in the overweight participants in my weight-management groups.

Even when they obviously do not have a weight problem, THE YOUNG ADULTS HAVE EATING PROBLEMS. I don't mean serious binge-and-purge problems, although that does occur occasionally. Frequently these young adults don't know where the fat in their diet is coming from. As I mentioned before, the typical meal in a school or college cafeteria, or in a fast-food restaurant, can contain 40 to 55 per cent or even more of its calories in fat. My students eat what they think is quite normal until they gain 5 or 10 pounds/2 to 5 kg. Then they go on a crash diet. Many of them never learn that fat makes you fat, and that there are many things you can eat to satisfy your appetite that won't make you fat. Of course, the more they diet the worse it gets, since repeated dieting makes it easier and easier to gain weight, and harder and harder to lose. In the end, many of them do become candidates for weight-control programmes!

With children and adolescents, WE DO NOT BELIEVE IN COUNTING ANYTHING, CALORIES OR FAT GRAMS.

We do believe in designing a healthy eating environment, and, at least in the home, you can do that. Of even greater importance, you can use the most powerful tool to encourage appropriate, healthy eating habits: YOUR *SILENT* EXAMPLE. When you adopt the T-Factor Diet, you, as a healthy model, provide the strongest incentive for all your family members to improve their eating habits.

Except for certain nutrients, your children need the same diet as yourself. Children are growing, of course, and they need more of the nutrients essential for growth. Unfortunately, many children have diets that are deficient in calcium, iron, vitamins A and C and the B vitamins.

Your children also need more calories than you do per pound of body weight, because they are growing, *but in a society where food is freely available you can forget about the extra growth calories*. Just provide a healthy eating environment and let your children's appetites determine their food intake.

Here are some general recommendations derived from the Basic Four Food Guide recommended by many American experts in childhood nutrition that will make sure your children receive all they need for growth and good health, and will not suffer from the dietary deficiencies (in calcium, iron, vitamins A and C and the B vitamins) I mentioned above.

Your children should have a wide variety of foods from each of the four food groups each day: (1) low-fat milk products; (2) lean meat, fish, or poultry; (3) vegetables and fruits; and (4) breads and cereals. Recommendations include:

4 servings of low-fat milk products
2 or more servings of lean meat, fish, or poultry
4 or more servings of vegetables and fruits, including one citrus fruit and a green or yellow vegetable
4 or more servings of breads and cereals (whole- or mixed-grain preferred).*

Notice the 'or more' suggestions in these recommendations, especially in vegetables, fruits and grain products. Children aged from four to ten generally require from 1,700 to 2,100 calories per day, and adolescents from eleven to seventeen generally require from 2,100 to 2,800 calories per day. The actual amount depends primarily on their increasing age, height, and weight, as well as level of physical activity.

---

* Obviously a serving size for a four-year-old is smaller than that for a seventeen-year-old but, in general, when we use the word 'serving' we refer to a standard cafeteria-size portion.

HOWEVER, AS I SAID BEFORE, WE DO NOT BELIEVE IN COUNTING ANYTHING, CALORIES OR FAT GRAMS.

Counting makes me nervous!

I don't mind counting when I'm in a research project, and Jamie Pope-Cordle and I both counted fat grams when we adopted the T-Factor Diet because we needed to change *faulty* eating patterns and we had no one but ourselves to take charge of our eating environments. Until you learn where the fat in your food is, and in the foot you serve your family, you, too, need to count fat grams. But counting encourages obsessional behaviour, and we want healthy eating to become second nature, as it did with us, and as it will for you, too, after only a few weeks.

Once you learn the fat contents of the various foods you want to include in the diet that you and your family eat we think it best to allow your children to determine what and how much they want to eat of everything you keep in your house. *You, however, have the responsibility to determine what's offered at home, and the manner in which it is served.* Remember: THE T-FACTOR DIET FOR CHILDREN AND ADOLESCENTS IS A FAMILY AFFAIR.

It is simply not fair to ask your children to do anything you aren't willing to do yourself when it comes to healthy eating. With prea-dolescent children, just do it. It doesn't take any negotiation. Get rid of the junk. Stock up on all the things you feel free to eat, and say, 'If you're hungry, just go to the cupboard or refrigerator and have anything you want.'

With adolescents, well, we've got a problem. (Who hasn't?)

If you have an overweight adolescent, it takes a kind of mutual non-aggression pact.

Adolescents are trying to establish their own identities and make the long transition to independence. They need to. (Do you really want your kids to stay at home all their lives?) If you have an overweight child who has reached the age of twelve or more, seek your opportunity. If, when you see an unhappy expression on your child's face, you ask, in a sympathetic way, 'What's wrong, darling?' and your child says that he or she is tired of being called a fatty, you've got your opening. That's when you can tell them the story about dietary fat and how to avoid it, *and show them all the good things to eat that are left*. Adolescents, just like everyone else, need to be able to eat when they are hungry and they are likely to be hungrier than adults simply because they are growing. Volunteer to set up the kind of home eating environment that will help them to achieve their ambition to be thin. Just look back at Tables 3.1 and 3.2 and choose the kinds of food you want to have in the house for snacks (we make some specific recommendations for children in Table 9.1 below). Go over the menus in Chapter Three and the recipes in

TABLE 9.1
SMART SNACKING FOR YOUR KIDS

Because 60 to 80 per cent of the calories in many snack foods are in the form of fat, it is a good idea to encourage healthy snack foods as early in life as possible. The following chart contains some of our suggestions.

Milk and Dairy Products	Low-fat or non-fat yoghurt mixed with fruit; low-fat cottage cheese or ricotta; other cheeses in moderate amounts; low-fat frozen yoghurt, hot cocoa made with skimmed or semi-skimmed milk; sorbets; puddings made with skimmed or semi-skimmed milk.
Vegetables	Fresh, crisp, cut-up raw vegetables with yoghurt-based dips; offer a variety of colours, shapes and sizes; keep in iced water in refrigerator for a quick crunch
Fruit	Fresh or dried fruit, frozen or slushy fruit (putting fruit in the freezer, such as bananas and grapes, makes a chilly summertime treat), fruit mixed with no- or low-fat yoghurt or milk; jellies made with fruit or skimmed milk
Breads and Cereals	Dry cereals, pretzels, popcorn, wholegrain pitta bread with vegetables or lean meats/cheese; wholegrain breads or rolls spread with low-fat cottage or ricotta cheese and jam, rice cakes, whole-grain crispbreads, bread sticks, muffins, currant loaf
Beverages	Water, fruit juices, home-made lemonade, skimmed or semi-skimmed milk, soda or mineral water, hot cocoa, herb and flower teas

Chapter Six and decide which foods will form the foundation for your family meals at home. REMEMBER THAT 80 PER CENT OF OBESE CHILDREN BECOME OBESE ADULTS! The decisions and choices you make when given this opportunity are likely to affect your children for the rest of their lives.

ADDITIONAL TIPS FOR EVERY DAY AND EVERYWHERE

You cannot control your child's entire eating environment, so don't try. Just controlling the home environment is half the battle and that may be all that is necessary.

Here is what our Vanderbilt Weight Management Program participant did to change her home environment and help her son to reduce his trouser size.

She got rid of all the high-fat biscuits, crisps and chocolate bars and replaced them with low-fat crispbreads, pretzels, rice cakes and fresh dried fruit (see Table 9.1 for specific suggestions).

She replaced the peanut butter in the teatime snack of peanut butter, toast and milk with apple butter.

She began to use only low-fat cuts of meat, prepared as I suggest in Chapter Six (and her family has not even noticed the change since everything tastes just as good as or better than before).

Instead of the chocolate and fudge or toffee that contain a major part of calories in fat, she has substituted plain boiled sweets or peppermints. In this way no one feels deprived. (Obviously we don't want children to overindulge on sugar for a variety of health reasons, but we have found that most people, including children, turn off after a maximum of about 100 calories in sugar sweets. That's a far cry from the 240 calories in a single 1.65 oz/40 g chocolate bar, of which 50 to 60 per cent of the calories come from fat. And when it comes to chocolate, it's not hard to eat 3 or 4 oz/80 or 100 g at a time.)

Here are some additional suggestions for dealing with the home environment, school, fast-food establishments and exercise:

- Find out what is offered at school if your child has lunches there and give advice on the lower-fat food choices.
- Pack a healthy lunch whenever possible (yes, it's more trouble, but why wait until your child is even fatter, or becomes a fat adult, and then have even greater problems?).
- If your child eats at any fast-food establishments, check them out, get nutritional information on the foods they serve, and advise your child on the best choices. If any of your child's

friends are also concerned about weight, this is a good time to get some peer cooperation.

- If possible, children should carry appropriate snack foods (such as fruit or low-fat crispbreads) whenever they have to be away from the house for long periods.
- Offer lots of love and support rather than nagging or criticizing your child about his or her weight.
- Cultivate a positive, healthy attitude towards foods and eating. The enjoyment of good, health-giving food is an important part of a satisfying life.
- Set a good example in the foods you choose and the amounts you consume – both at home and away.
- Try new foods, be adventurous, but don't force these new foods on your children. Let them help themselves to a small portion. Young children are especially sensitive to strong tastes or extremes of temperature or texture, but don't forever banish a food that has been once refused, because taste buds change.
- Establish dependable mealtimes. This helps to regulate your child's appetite and lends some structure to the day – which facilitates a sense of security.
- Small children have relatively high energy needs, so, since their stomachs cannot hold a lot of food at one time, include at least two snacks a day in addition to meals.
- Do not force children to finish everything on their plates when their appetites are satisfied with less.
- Don't forbid 'junk food', but don't keep it in the house all the time. If you believe that all your child will eat is junk food, think about who is buying it!
- Don't use food as a reward or as a pacifier.
- Provide a safe environment for your child to run and play.
- Don't carry a child who can walk.
- Make your daily routine and your child's more active by walking more and driving less.
- Ration television time. A child glued to the tube is a child not being active (and there is a direct relationship between the number of hours spent watching TV as a child and adolescent obesity).
- Encourage your child to play outdoors throughout the year. Simply wrap them up well when the weather is cold or wet.
- Share enjoyable, physical activities with your child. Plan family walks, bike rides and other active outings.
- Encourage your child to play with other children.
- Plan active family vacations, reinforcing the idea that exercise is fun and worth pursuing.
- Give an older child responsibility for exercising the family pet.

SOME FINAL ADVICE

Unless your child is severely obese, most experts do not suggest that you make any effort to reduce his or her weight. It is much better to encourage healthy eating habits such as we have designed in the T-Factor Diet, and let the slightly overweight child grow into his or her adult weight.

However, if you feel that your child is seriously overweight, consult your school or family doctor for assessment and recommendations or referral. Some of the commercial organizations such as Weight Watchers will give teenagers – boys as well as girls – supportive help.

CHAPTER TEN

MYTHS AND MYSTERIES OF WEIGHT MANAGEMENT

IF YOU CRAVE CARBOHYDRATES YOU'D BETTER SATISFY THAT CRAVING!

A great deal has been written about carbohydrate cravings. If you think that you suffer from some abnormality in this respect because you seem always to crave something sweet, you've probably been given conflicting and confusing advice. Some experts think of carbohydrate cravings as some sort of malady that requires a cure, while others advise satisfying such cravings with totally inappropriate foods, such as a bag of sweets.

The truth about carbohydrate cravings is that changes in the body's small store of carbohydrate energy (the glycogen stores) exert a powerful influence on appetite. This influence is much stronger than changes in the much larger fat stores and demands satisfaction.

Since the body only stores about 2,000 calories in glycogen and tends generally to burn it over a twenty-four-hour period in equal proportion to fat, it is quite easy for the body to turn over half or more of its glycogen storage every day. In contrast, only about 1 per cent or less of the total fat storage may be affected since our bodies may easily store 100,000 calories or more as fat. If the glycogen stores are not replenished in that day's diet as the energy is drained from them to support our activities, the impact is felt immediately.

Experiments with laboratory animals show that a decrease in the intake of carbohydrate on one day results in an immediate increase in food intake on the next. The reverse is true when more carbohydrate is eaten than is burned in the fuel mixture. That is, when

191

animals overeat on carbohydrate, they eat less the next day. With fat, on the other hand, there seems to be an unfortunate snowball effect: for some unexplained reason, high fat consumption on a given day seems to lead to continued increased fat consumption on the subsequent day!

Many variables affect appetite. Some we are all acutely conscious of, such as the sight and smell of tasty foods, which turn on a physiological readiness to eat. However, your body's glycogen stores exert one of the most potent physiological regulators of appetite. The influence is not as direct or as easily recognized as the sight of food or the pangs of an empty stomach, but the impact is almost irresistible. You *will* become ravenous if you do not take in enough carbohydrate to meet the body's daily demand for glucose in its fuel mixture.

For example, if you've been accustomed to skipping breakfast and having a light lunch in an effort to control your food intake, only to find yourself almost out of control from 5 p.m. until you go to bed, it's probably because you have depleted half your glycogen stores and messages are pouring in from every cell in your body, like hundreds of Jewish grandmothers crying 'EAT, EAT!'

And eat you should.

In fact, you would have been better off if you had been eating all day long, nibbling on the carbohydrate foods that would have kept your glycogen stores near maximum. Although many nutritionists still recommend eating 'three square meals' without snacks, that approach is really not the most natural to humankind. It was much more natural to us throughout the long course of our evolutionary history to nibble on whatever was available, usually grains, fruits or vegetables, whenever we felt the slightest bit hungry. One of the best ways to avoid the development of the 'hidden hunger' which suddenly appears to overwhelm you after a period of deprivation and leads to overeating (if not bingeing) is to eat whenever the urge hits you.

But you must eat the right foods – that is, the kinds of foods that were available to your ancient ancestors.

Unfortunately, the right foods are frequently hard to come by when you need them. I'm talking about fresh fruit and vegetables, and wholegrain breads and cereals, with little or no fat content. These are the foods that can regulate glycogen storage without contributing to fat storage. Processed snack foods have been made more attractive to most people than natural foods, they have been scientifically formulated with added fat combined with sugar and salt to satisfy natural flavour preferences (which I'll discuss later in this chapter) beyond the ability of naturally occurring foods to do so. As a result when you try to satisfy your carbohydrate cravings with anything but naturally occurring foods you end up with fat you really don't need. Let me give you just a few examples. Over 60 per cent of the calories in most crisps and chocolate bars come from fat, while only 30 to 35 per cent are carbohydrate; the cheese sandwich biscuits that people sometimes choose as an alternative to sweets for a quick snack also generally contain over 60 per cent of calories from fat, with only 25 per cent of calories from carbohydrate.

Think for a moment about what this can mean if you have a weight problem. Suppose you are down a couple of hundred glycogen calories. The 240-calorie chocolate bar or packet of crisps contains only 50 to 75 carbohydrate calories, the rest is fat. The fat will end up in your fat cells and you will still not have satisfied your glycogen needs. You will be hungry again shortly and likely to overeat at meals because you have not satisfied these glycogen needs. You will get fatter and fatter because you keep on taking in more fat calories than you can burn in your daily fuel mixture, all as a result of an unconscious striving to satisfy your body's natural and healthy drive to replenish glycogen.

I hope you see the point. It bears much repetition and it must sink in! If you choose a food that contains fat in addition to carbohydrate when your appetite has beens stimulated by glycogen depletion, you add fat to your fat stores before you get enough carbohydrate to satisfy your legitimate carbohydrate craving. (I discuss the reasons for our fatty food preferences below.)

The T-Factor solution to carbohydrate cravings is to make sure that the majority of calories at all meals comes from carbohydrate, not fat, and to reach for a carbohydrate whenever you are hungry for a snack. You may find that this eliminates cravings completely; it is certainly the only way to satisfy them. Since your body has such a limited ability to convert carbohydrate to fat, there is a built-in protection against putting on weight when you satisfy carbohydrate cravings with real carbohydrate foods rather than fatty foods.*

* Glycogen depletion sets up such a demand for satisfaction that nature seems to have built in a protection against long-term discomfort. People on a fast report how hunger seems to lessen and sometimes almost disappear after twenty-four to forty-eight hours. In part this may be due to the body's ability to switch its fuel requirements to near total fat during a fast, and to produce waste products in the form of ketones, which diminish appetite. Other changes occur with fasting that increase the body's ability to store fat so that once a fasting person starts to eat again, it is easier to gain weight and become fatter than before the fast.

SET POINT: THE POINT THAT ISN'T A POINT

One of the most unfortunate misconceptions to have been foisted on the overweight public is the notion of a set point. It's unfortunate not only because it is a discouraging concept, but because it's simply wrong.

The term 'set point' has been used to describe the body's apparent preference for a certain weight or amount of body fat. It implies a self-correcting mechanism whereby attempts to change weight or fat storage are met with counterforces that are designed to return you to 'THE set point' and defeat any diet or weight-reducing plan.

There are certainly strong genetic influences on body-fat storage. It becomes obvious when anyone compares his or her body build with that of a similarly built ancestor who also deposited fat in identical parts of the body and had a weight problem! In addition, the easy and almost unlimited availability of fatty foods turns on our appetite and constantly tempts us to return to a pattern of high fat intake. As I've explained before, your excess body fat results from eating more fat in your diet than the amount you burn each day in your fuel mixture. This means that when you combine a given heritage with a given life-style – that is, a certain amount of fat in the diet and a certain amount of exercise – you get a certain body weight.

But there is no such thing as *a* set point! There are, in reality, many set points. Speaking from a biological perspective, there is *a range of adaptability* within which permanent changes in diet and exercise operate with a certain ease and convenience. The range comprises about 3½–5 stone (22–34 kg).

If you eat a diet that contains 40 per cent or more of its calories in fat and you do no regular fat-burning exercises, you are likely to drift up to the top of your range of adaptability. That is, you may end up weighing perhaps as much as 5 stone (34 kg) more than necessary.

But you don't have to stay there! If you reduce your fat intake and engage in this kind of exercise that burns a few hundred FAT CALORIES each day, you will drift down to the bottom of your range of adaptability and lose whatever excess weight you have gained – PERMANENTLY.

To put it another way, when you follow the T-Factor Diet and Activity Programme you adjust your 'set point' to its lowest level and it stays there!

Obviously, if you want to weigh even 5 pounds (2 kg) more or less than what you weigh today, for ever, you must do something different in the way of your diet or exercise, for ever. Both diet and exercise are important, and the T-Factor programme makes the necessary changes livable and enjoyable. Exercise, however, may prove to provide the heretofore elusive key. I have already discussed the major role it can play from physiological and psychological standpoints in Chapters Seven and Eight. In addition, a recent research study that compared sedentary and active people showed that exercise may naturally and automatically change your dietary preferences away from fatty foods to carbohydrates. I think you will find that this is likely to occur for you, too, for two reasons. First, carbohydrate foods tend to contain much more water than fatty foods, and people who exercise find an increased appetite for foods that can replace the water they lose while exercising. Second, even if you concentrate on fat-burning exercise, any exercise at all will deplete glycogen stores beyond the level reached by a sedentary person, and this is likely to increase your appetite for carbohydrate foods.

WHY DO HUMAN BEINGS SEEM TO HAVE A PREFERENCE FOR HIGH-FAT FOODS?

Although glycogen depletion provides a strong internal signal that turns on appetite, human beings seem to turn to *fatty* carbohydrate foods to satisfy that appetite if those foods are present in the environment. The urge to eat fatty carbohydrates, preferably sweetened or salted, has a long evolutionary history and was cultivated as a resistance to famine and infectious disease.

Ever since the human race turned from hunting and gathering to agriculture for its food supply, we have faced frequent famines. In fact, two-thirds of the earth's population still faces serious food shortages every two years or so. Only in the Western world, and only for the past few hundred years, has there been anything approaching a stable food supply. Genetic lines that tended to store body fat, and that developed a preference for foods that could put down fat fast (considering that the food supply might be here today and gone tomorrow) were favoured under these boom-or-bust conditions.

Infectious disease played a similar selective role. Together with famine, infectious disease often prevented half the newborn infants from reaching their first birthday. Before antibiotics and immunization, resistance to infectious disease depended in part on the amount of body fat an individual possessed, since the metabolic rate goes up about 7 per cent for each degree of fever. With just a slight rise in normal body temperature, energy needs are about 28 per cent greater than normal. Thus, individuals with a genetic tendency to obesity, or who liked fatty foods and had laid down a few extra pounds of fat storage, would be more likely to survive.

Because in the past individuals who did not possess the capacity to store fat easily or who did not care for fatty foods had less of a chance to reach reproductive age, we tend to be a species with rather strong tendencies to obesity given the availability of high-fat foods. Indeed, just the sight of such foods (not counting the smell and anticipated taste) starts the flow of saliva and gastric juices and turns on our appetite.

Of course, enterprising food manufacturers capitalize on this natural tendency and design 'unnatural' foods that will stimulate our appetites even more than anything found in nature. Knowing the preference for fat, salt and sweetness, scientists can design 'super-natural' foods which blend these characteristics and turn on appetite beyond our needs for survival. The appetites of almost all human beings turn off before they can overeat on apples or other fruits, vegetables and grains, but not before they overeat on chocolate bars, crisps and other snack foods. Millions of dollars are spent developing such foods, because if we didn't come to prefer them over apples and oranges, these food manufacturers would have a difficult time showing any profits.

Which brings me to a discussion of the role of behaviour modification and the reasons for its rather poor showing as a tool in weight management.

LEARNING FROM FAILURE: WHAT CAN BEHAVIOUR MODIFICATION DO FOR YOU?

It's been about twenty years since behaviour modification techniques were first applied to weight management and the best that can be said is that they help participants in formal weight-management programmes lose an average of about 10–12 pounds (4–5 kg), and that only a small minority is able to keep that weight off for more than one year.

Why?

In theory, the more you apply behaviour modification techniques, the more you learn about controlling your eating behaviour and the easier it should become. In practice, it doesn't work this way, as I'm sure you know if you have ever been in a behaviour modification programme for weight control. Behaviour modification techniques are a bore and a bother. There is a limit to the extent most people are willing to continue keeping eating records, putting their forks down between bites, eating from tiny dishes and thinking up artificial, insignificant rewards for controlling their eating behaviour. The force of social and emotional pressures to overeat on fatty foods is in the end much greater than any reward or punishment that we can control in a free society!

In my opinion, there is only one behaviour modification element that can help you when your normal environment is forever tempting you with super-natural fatty foods that turn on your appetite beyond your needs for energy – AVOIDANCE. I know of no behaviour modification strategy that can forever protect you from the innate biological predisposition that stimulates appetite when you see, smell or even imagine the taste of your particular favourite high-fat foods if they are all readily available! You cannot deny Mother Nature for ever, you will succumb.

So the only behaviour modification strategy that has a chance of helping you is: CHANGE YOUR ENVIRONMENT.

The commonest response from successful people who are asked what change they made in their eating behaviour is: 'I keep junk food out of the house.' They do not indicate that they aim for total denial – they occasionally plan a 'mini-binge' and enjoy it. *But they customarily AVOID temptation.*

There are a few other ways, however, in which behaviour modification techniques may be applied in combination T-Factor Diet principles to provide you with greater success than ever before.

Normally, behaviourists suggest that you find alternative activities whenever eating urges that appear to be greater than your daily energy strike. That is still a good idea especially if you turn to physical activity. Remember, however, that eating urges often arise from glycogen depletion after you have restrained yourself from eating a nutritious breakfast or lunch. Try my suggestions for breakfast and lunch, and then, SO LONG AS YOU DON'T EAT FATTY FOODS, THERE ARE PLENTY OF GOOD THINGS TO EAT WHENEVER YOU FEEL LIKE MUNCHING.

The most important thing you can learn when it comes to your eating behaviour is that, so long as you don't exceed the guidelines for fat consumption, you are likely to be able to eat whenever you wish without harming your efforts at weight-control.

Our research also shows that social pressures, especially at parties and in restaurants, frequently lead to overeating on high-fat foods. One of the best ways to erase the social pressure is to get as many as possible of the people who interact with you on a daily basis to adopt the T-Factor Diet and start eating in a more nutritious fashion. Once you are all eating in a more nutritious way, it is easier to 'save up' for the special occasions, and to return the next day to your basic T-Factor Diet.*

Finally, a certain percentage of those who overeat on high-fat foods do so for emotional reasons. After all, when you're feeling down, you don't run to the refrigerator for a carrot. There is something about fatty sweets or fatty salty snacks that is particularly satisfying. The reasons for this are not entirely clear, but some experts feel it has something to do with the impact of fatty foods on the endorphins. In some people, fatty foods may stimulate pleasurable feelings via changes in this or some other hormone secretion.

If you feel that you overeat for emotional reasons, I think you should look for specific help in solving the emotional problems that stimulate your appetite. Learning to deal with that life situation will provide a more satisfactory and more permanent solution than letting the problems continue and trying to find substitutes for eating. But I do have one suggestion: There are plenty of good things to eat on the T-Factor Diet whenever you have an urge to eat for any reason. To be specific, if you haven't learned how to deal with people who aggravate you, you're much better off chewing on a wholemeal roll when you feel like biting their heads off than you are downing a packet of crisps or a bag of doughnuts.

WHY IS IT SO EASY TO GAIN WEIGHT AFTER FASTING OR USING A LOW-CALORIE FORMULA DIET, AND WHAT CAN YOU DO ABOUT IT?

One way to increase your body's ability to gain weight and to encourage higher levels of fat storage is to fast or to use a low-calorie formula diet (600 calories or less per day) for a prolonged period of time. Unfortunately – perhaps out of frustration with the poor results obtained with moderate calorie-reduced diets – many respected health professionals are beginning to encourage the low-calorie formula diets for people 50 pounds (20 kg) or more over desirable weight. While there are certainly some instances where such dieting is called for because of medical reasons to lose weight quickly, there are far too many people for whom such dieting will prove counterproductive.

---

* Other suggestions for choosing nutritious foods when eating out will be found in Chapter Four, where experiences of people on the T-Factor Diet are recounted.

In my opinion there are many more people who will end up heavier than ever before after using these diets than there are people who will lose weight and keep it off.

There are two important reasons for avoiding low-calorie formula diets unless called for in a medical emergency.

First, there is a severe reduction in metabolic rate. It averages about 25 per cent and can reach as high as 40 per cent. While the proponents of the formula diets claim that there is 'on average' a return to normal after the diet, there is evidence to show that a certain percentage of users may not return to normal, even after a considerable period of time.

Second, after several weeks on a formula diet, when you start eating again there is a rebound in the activity of the fat-incorporating enzyme, adipose tissue lipoprotein lipase. This enzyme controls the rate at which fat is entered into your fat cells and that rate may be elevated 300 or 400 per cent above normal. It's as though the fat is being sucked right out of the bloodstream and soaked up by your fat cells. At least one study has shown that this elevation may last for a year after the diet, and only return to normal or to near-normal levels *once you have regained all your weight*.

Some years ago, following another period of great enthusiasm over these formula diets, I had former users of one popular formula who were having trouble maintaining their weight keep daily eating records for me. Months after losing weight on their formula diet, we found that the women were likely to gain weight whenever they exceeded 1,200 calories per day, while the one man in the group gained weight on 1,500 calories. This helped explain why people who had lost weight on a formula diet only to regain it were among the hardest to help in any subsequent efforts to lose weight.

There are both principled and unprincipled persons in the business of selling low-calorie formula diets. If you feel you must use such drastic measures to lose weight in spite of my belief that you can deal with the problem in a much simplier, healthier, and less expensive way with the T-Factor Diet, the best programmes require your agreement to participate in long-term follow-up and nutritional counselling, with payment in advance to assure commitment. The persons in charge appreciate the tremendous difficulty you will face keeping your weight off after the diet and, rather than just sell their product, where most of the profit lies, they employ a staff of health professionals at a much smaller profit to offer group and personal counselling in order to increase their success rate. *Don't ever consider using a formula diet unless you are willing to make a commitment to the follow-up programme.*

If you have ever used a formula diet and now find that it is harder to maintain your weight than ever before, stop thinking calories, start thinking fat grams, and engage in fat-burning physical activity every day! In view of your body's eagerness to refill its fat stores, your best chance of managing your weight lies in controlling your fat intake at the lower levels of the T-Factor Diet. If you are presently using a formula diet, be sure to increase fat intake very slowly when you enter the refeeding phase because there is likely to be a preferential shunting of fat to storage rather than to direct energy use after the diet. That is, you are likely to gain a lot of weight even if you eat very little fat. And remember that if you fail to exercise and you allow total calorie intake to exceed your energy needs every day, you may even force the conversion of carbo-hydrate to fat.

EPILOGUE

Compared with the also-rans, champions in all human activities seem to have a cognitive environment that is quite different. They have the highest standards and they have complete confidence that if they follow certain rules, they will reach them. If you could crawl inside their heads, you would hear them say these rules over and over again and you would hear mainly positive conversations with themselves. As a result, when you observe their behaviour you see that it is focused and that they work hard to reach their goals.

Here are the kinds of statement that should be flowing around in your head. Let them become rules for you. Practise attaching their meanings to your behaviour – that is, SAY these things over and over again as you DO them, and you will never be fat again.

ONLY FAT MAKES ME FAT.

I EAT ANYTHING I WANT EXCEPT FOR FATTY FOODS.

I AM AN ACTIVE PERSON.

DOING IS KNOWING.

I CAN BECOME GOOD AT ANYTHING I WANT IF I PRACTISE EVERY DAY.

EVERY TIME I GO FOR A WALK I LEAVE SOME FAT IN MY FOOTSTEPS.

A LOW-FAT DINNER MAKES ME THINNER.

MY TUMMY STAYS FLAT WHEN I DON'T EAT FAT.

I'M FIT, NOT FAT.

JACK SPRAT COULD EAT NO FAT, WHICH IS WHY HE
WEIGHED 4 STONE LESS THAN MRS SPRAT.

APPENDIX A

ADDITIONAL SCIENTIFIC BACKGROUND FOR THE T-FACTOR DIET

Several years ago, certain leading biochemists and physiologists began investigating whether increasing the ratio of carbohydrate to fat in the diet could make a difference in the prevalence of obesity (Danforth, 1985). Based on evidence (already outlined in Chapter Two) that fat is more easily accumulated in the body from dietary fat than from carbohydrate, Danforth concluded that, based on theoretical grounds, an increased ratio of carbohydrate to fat in the diet could make a difference, even if total caloric intake remains the same. The metabolic cost of convering carbohydrate for energy use or storage in the human body is much greater than that of converting fat. Thus, many of the calories contained in carbohydrate foods are simply wasted and given off as heat rather than put to useful work or stored within the body. In addition – and this may be of even greater importance – the body appears to have limited ability to convert carbohydrate to fat even after consuming carbohydrate loads far greater than one would spontaneously consume (Flatt, 1987).

In one of the earlier studies on this latter issue, Acheson, Flatt and Jequier (1982) fed a group of six men a meal containing 500 grams (2,000 calories) of carbohydrate. During the next ten hours they found that only 9 grams of fat (81 calories) were produced from the carbohydrate in this meal, and that their subjects went into negative fat balance. That is, the fuel mixture being burned during those ten hours required more fat than could be converted from the carbohydrate in the meal, and this fat had to be withdrawn from tissue storage of fat.

In another study, Acheson et al. (1984) tested the impact of a 2,000-calorie carbohydrate load on subjects who had been acclimatized to three different diets: a high-fat diet, a standard mixed diet, and a high-carbohydrate diet. On the high-fat diet, glycogen stores were reduced and one would not expect that much of the carbohydrate would be turned to fat since the first priority in the body would be to replenish the depleted glycogen. On the high-carbohydrate diet one might expect considerable conversion of carbohydrate to fat, since the glycogen stores were already quite full. Nevertheless, once again, only about 81 calories of fat were produced from the 2,000-calorie carbohydrate load even when the subjects had been eating a high-carbohydrate diet. And again, they went into negative fat balance. In addition, Acheson et al. found that the higher the carbohydrate content of the customary diet, the greater the thermic effect of the single meal, which illustrates the greater thermogenic potential of high-carbohydrate compared with high-fat diets.

In a third study, which I have previously mentioned in Chapter Two, Flatt et al. (1985) varied the fat content of a breakfast containing a set amount of protein and carbohydrate. On each of two days the breakfast contained about 120 calories of protein and about 292 calories of carbohydrate. On one day it contained about 54 calories in fat, and on the other day it contained about 414 calories in fat. On both days, the amount of protein and carbohydrate used in the fuel mixture over the next nine hours very closely approximated the amount contained in the breakfast. That is, all the protein and carbohydrate energy in the breakfast was burned, but on both days, regardless of the fat in the breakfast, the body burned about 360 calories of fat in its fuel mixture. Thus, on the high-fat day there was fat left over for storage, whereas on the low-fat day about 300 calories in fat were withdrawn from fat storage.

It is possible to force the body to convert a portion of dietary carbohydrate to fat after sustained large excesses of carbohydrate in the diet. However, before such conversion takes place it is necessary to maximize the body's ability to store glycogen. In a recent study, Acheson et al. (1988) used a combination of exercise and diet first to deplete glycogen stores and then to saturate them on a high-carbohydrate diet. Each day, in order to saturate glycogen stores, they fed their subjects 1,500 more calories than they had burned on the previous day. Before an appreciable conversion of carbohydrate to fat took place, there was a massive increase in glycogen storage until considerably higher than normal levels were reached (an average of 810 grams of glycogen storage versus the more usual average of about 500 grams). In addition, there was a 35 per cent increase in the metabolic rate so that by Day 7 of overfeeding in the experiment (the last day of overfeeding) the subjects were consuming over 5,000 calories a day, approximately 4,000 of which were in the form of carbohydrate. This represented a diet-induced increase in energy requirements (adaptive thermogenesis) of about 1,400 calories per day (up from about 3,600 on the second day of the overfeeding to 5,000 on the seventh) in order to maintain that surplus of 1,500 calories above the previous day's energy needs. On the second day of overfeeding by 1,500 calories, thee was a fat conversion from carbohydrate of about 270 calories and on the fourth day it reached 720 calories. The researchers estimated that thereafter some 70 to 75 per cent of the excess intake would be retained in fat storage.

Acheson and his colleagues concluded that while it is possible to force the conversion of carbohydrate to fat, to do so glycogen stores must first increase by about 500 grams over their normal level (about 2,000 calories over normal). That is, the body can handle periodic loads of 2,000 calories of carbohydrate without contributing to fat synthesis and storage. In order to continue appreciable conversion of carbohydrate to fat, continued massive amounts of carbohydrate over and above daily energy needs, such as they used in their study, would have to be ingested.

When it comes to weight control, the moral of this last study seems to be that while excess dietary fat is easily converted to fat storage, excess carbohydrate is not. Thus, if you want to pig-out occasionally with little danger of gaining fat weight, do it on carbohydrates.

There is one other point worth mentioning with respect to weight control on a high-carbohydrate diet, however, and that is the likelihood of rather large swings in one's daily weight. Since fluctuations in carbohydrate intake within the 2,000-calorie (500-gram) range mentioned above have a direct impact on glycogen stores, rather than fat stores, and since glycogen is stored at around 500 calories per pound/450 g of body weight due to its solution of 1 part glycogen to 3 to 4 parts water, daily variations in carbohydrate intake can easily cause swings of a pound or two. This is really the weight of the water in solution, and it goes down as easily as it goes up. (Fat variations are not as easily detectable on a daily basis because the body stores fat at around 3,500 calories per pound. And, once gained, fat weight, as we all know, does not go down as easily as water weight!)

BODY COMPOSITION IS ADJUSTED TO FAT IN THE DIET

In the steady state, where one is not gaining or losing body fat, the proportion of carbohydrate and fat in the fuel mixture powering the body each day is equal to the proportion of carbohydrate and fat in the diet. If one eats more fat than is being burned each day, it is put into fat storage and the fat reserves increase to the point where energy needs, as a function of increased body weight and increased fat stores, match the intake. At a new higher weight, with greater fat storage, the fat used in the fuel mix reaches the level of the fat in the high-fat diet. As Flatt (1987) pointed out, 'On diets with a relatively high fat content (such as the mixed diets consumed in affluent societies), a substantial expansion of the adipose [fat] tissue mass often occurs before the use of fat reaches a rate commensurate with the diet's fat content.' And furthermore: 'Obesity may be the result of a tendency to achieve the steady state, where the fuel mix oxidized has the same composition as the food consumed only after an undesirably large expansion of the adipose tissue mass has taken place'.

The relationship of the body's fat composition to the nature of the diet is being disclosed in a rash of recent studies. The relationship is easiest to illustrate in animals because of our ability to control the diet in laboratory research. In one study, with mice as subjects, as fat intake increased from 1 to 65 per cent of calories, obesity increased from 0 to 35 per cent. In the range of 20 to 40 per cent of daily calories from fat, which pretty much includes the lower and upper ends of the range we are concerned with in humans, body-fat content *doubled* (Salmon and Flatt, 1985).

Of the human studies, a recent report using data that assessed dietary intake over a one-year period from the Nurses Health Study showed that there was no relationship between total energy intake and obesity in a group of 141 women aged thirty-four to fifty-nine (Romieu et al., 1988). There was, however, a significant relationship between fat intake (specifically saturated-fat intake) and obesity. These authors also noted a strong relationship between lack of physical activity (such as distances walked and stairs climbed each day) and obesity.

IMPACT OF A LOW-FAT DIET ON BODY WEIGHT IN HUMANS

There have been several studies in which a low-fat diet was recommended in connection with certain medical problems. Although weight loss was *not* a specific objective, it seemed to occur naturally.

In one study (Asp et al., 1987), as part of their treatment for breast cancer, a group of seventeen women reduced their total fat intake from 39 per cent of total calories to 22 per cent. Over a three-month period they lost approximately 6.5 pounds. While weight loss was not an objective, the increase in bulk of the diet was associated with a lowering of total calories, from approximately 1,840 at the start of the change in diet to approximately 1,375 at the conclusion. Total daily fat intake went down from about 80 grams, which is quite typical of a North American diet, to about 35 grams, which is within the range I recommend on the T-Factor Diet.

A team of investigators at the Division of Nutritional Sciences at Cornell University (Lissnet et al., 1987) examined weight changes in twenty-four women who rotated for two-week periods between diets containing 15–20, 30–35, or 45–50 per cent of the energy derived from fat. The diets were designed to be equally palatable (although the subjects tended to prefer the low-fat diet) and the women could eat as much of anything as they desired. On the low-fat diet they consumed approximately 2,087 calories per day and lost almost a pound/450 g each week.* On the high-fat diet they consumed about 2,714 calories and gained about 11 ounces/300 g each week. They maintained their weight on the medium-fat diet, consuming about 2,352 calories per day. The low-fat diet, on which the subjects lost weight on over 2,000 calories per day, contained on average under 40 grams of fat. The women in this study were maintaining weight on about 98 grams of fat per day, while the high-fat diet, on which they gained weight, contained over 140 grams of fat per day. The amount of weight lost or gained each week corresponds almost exactly to the difference in the energy contained in the dietary fat that was subtracted or added to the maintenance diets. *Weight loss was inversely related to the total amount of carbohydrate and protein in the diet.* Total calories from protein and carbohydrates equalled about 1,722 on the low-fat diet and about 1,425 on the high-fat diet. In addition, the total weight of the food consumed on the low-fat diet was significantly higher than that on the high-fat diet.†

* Interestingly, while this study employed normal-weight subjects who used each of the diets for only two weeks, the weight loss achieved on the low-fat diet is approximately what overweight women using the T-Factor Diet obtained in the Vanderbilt Weight Management Program over periods as long as twenty weeks, with calorie intakes as high as 2,000 calories a day.

† On the low-, medium-, and high-fat diets, approximately 13, 12, and 10 per cent of calories was derived from protein, and approximately 70, 55, and 42 per cent of calories was derived from carbohydrate, respectively. Because of low energy density (in fruits, vegetables and grains) the weight and bulk of a high-carbohydrate diet are greater than those of a low-carbohydrate diet.

Finally, at the University of Alberta in Canada (Brown et al., 1984), a group of fifty average-weight men and women suffering from peripheral vascular disease were asked to follow either an American Heart Association (AHA) lipid-reducing diet or a higher-fibre, lower-fat version of the Pritikin maintenance diet (HFD). Subjects assigned to either diet benefited greatly, but those in the AHA group ended up twelve months later consuming about 34 per cent of their days' total average of 1,687 calories in fat, while the HFD group ended up consuming about 16 per cent of their days' total average of 1,608 calories in fat. In grams, this amounts to about 63 grams of fat per day in the AHA group, and about 28 grams of fat per day in the HFD group. Although the participants in this study were not overweight, the American Heart Association group lost an average of 9 pounds/265 g (from 113 per cent of average weight to 105 per cent), while the group asked to follow a higher-fibre, lower-fat diet lost over 13 pounds/385 g (from 109 per cent of average weight to 99 per cent). Once again, weight loss was inversely related total carbohydrate and protein consumption (average of 1,120 calories, carbohydrate and protein combined, in the AHA group, and 1,344 calories, combined, in the HFD group).

You might ask why the participants in these groups did not continue to lose weight indefinitely on a low-fat diet. In other words, how and when does stabilization occur? It works something like this:

When you switch from a high- to low-fat diet, your body pulls fat from your fat cells in order to maintain the present high proportion of fat to carbohydrate in its fuel mix. At the same time as you lose body fat and move towards some new, and lower, body-fat content, you begin to make gradual adjustments in your fuel mixture, moving towards matching the change in diet. When you reach stabilization at some new and lower weight, your fuel mix will now approximate the new dietary ratio of carbohydrate to fat.

Of course, no one can tell what the new weight and body-fat content will be in any individual case when he or she changes the fat content of the diet. You have to find out by experience.

You might also ask, on the basis of the results of the Canadian study, why I am not simply recommending a Pritikin maintenance diet, and the reason is quite easy to understand. Although the Pritikin program is based on what is essentially a good idea it is carried beyond the tolerance and endurance of very many people! Anyone who has tried the Pritikin program knows that it is a terribly restricted diet and very hard to maintain. Indeed, the subjects in the study I've just discussed were not able to stick with it. But, fortunately, with the modifications they spontaneously added to it, they ended up close enough to the total fat-gram target that I recommend in the T-Factor Diet to be illustrative of what you can expect when you cut total daily fat grams down to 20–40 for women and 30–60 for men.*

CONCLUSION

I have referred to a selection of the most pertinent studies illustrating the importance of the composition of the diet to energy balance and fat storage. For a more exhaustive review of the many factors involved in energy balance in human beings, see Sims (1986) as well as Danforth (1985) and Flatt (1987). The unique merits of a low-fat diet for weight control are fully discussed by McCarty (1986) in an article bearing that title. This article closes with an observation that makes the point quite nicely:

'Calorie counting' is one of the more grotesque manifestations of the modern American scene. While it may be useful for a small percentage of the stoic, highly motivated individuals, few fallible humans will submit to this rigorous discipline for a lifetime. The dismal long-term success rates of most weight-control programs bear witness to the futility of calorie counting as a weight-loss strategy. Calorie counters are usually doomed to failure because they continue to eat the fatty Western foods which made them fat in the first place – albeit in restricted quantities. Sooner or later their discipline fails, and their weight goes back up.

* As the type for this book was being set, a study appeared in the *American Journal of Clinical Nutrition*, 1989, 49, 77–85 by R. L. Hammer, C. A. Barrier, E. S. Roundy, J. M. Bradford, and A. G. Fisher: titled 'Calorie-restricted low-fat diet and exercise in obese women'.

In one experimental condition, subjects ate a low-fat, unrestricted carbohydrate diet, with no attempt to cut calories, and slowly increased their physical activity until they were able to walk or jog about 3 miles four or five days a week. The calorie and fat intake ended up matching almost exactly what we have been obtaining in clinical practice when we prescribe the T-Factor Diet in the Vanderbilt Program. The weight loss over 16 weeks was also almost identical, that is, almost a pound/450 g a week (14¾ pounds/6.7 k in 16 weeks). The authors reported that this approach to losing weight was well received by the participants, and the authors concluded, 'A low-fat, high-carbohydrate diet combined with daily exercise is effective in causing weight and fat loss in obese women without altering RMR [resting metabolic rate] and results in improved cardiovascular fitness', and, 'A program similar to the ALX [their ad libitum-carbohydrate diet with exercise] treatment is an effective prescription for weight and health management of obsese persons'.

Contrast that with the experience of many primitive groups whose traditional diets are low in fat. They have never heard of a 'calorie', they eat as much as they want, they get some exercise – and they remain slender throughout life. Here's a weight-control program with a *proven* track record!.

REFERENCES

Acheson, K. J., Flatt, J. P., and Jequier, E. (1952). Glycogen synthesis versus lipogenesis after a 500 gram carbohydrate meal in man. *Metabolism*, 31, 1234–1240.

Acheson, K. J., Schutz, Y., Bessard, T., Anantharaman, K., Flatt, J. P., and Jequier, E. (1988). Glycogen storage capacity and de novo lipogenesis curing massive carbohydrate overfeeding in man. *American Journal of Clinical Nutrition*, 48, 240–247.

Acheson, K. J., Schutz, Y., Bessard, T., Ravussin, E., and Jequier, E. (1984). Nutritional influences on lipogenesis and thermogenesis after a carbohydrate meal. *American Journal of Physiology*, 246, E62–70.

Asp, E. H., Buzzard, I. M., Chlebowski, R. T., Nixon, D., Blackburn, D., Jochimsen, P., Scanlon, E., Insull, W., Elashoff, R., Butrum, R., and Wynder, E. (1987). Reducing total fat intake: Effect on body weights, *International Journal of Obesity*, 4, 3979–3976.

Brown, G. D., Whyte, L., Gee, M. I., Crockford, P. M., Grace, M., Oberle, K., Williams, H. T. G., and Hutchinson, K. J. (1984). Effects of two 'lipid lowering' diets on plasma lipid levels of patients with peripheral vascular disease. *Journal of the American Dietetic Association*, 84, 546–550.

Danforth, E. (1985). Diet and obesity. *American Journal of Clinical Nutrition*, 41, 1132–1145.

Flatt, J. P. (1987). Dietary fat, carbohydrate balance, and weight maintenance: Effects of exercise. *American Journal of Clinical Nutrition*, 45, 296–306.

Flatt, J. P., Ravussin, E., Acheson, K. J., and Lequier, E. (1985). Effects of dietary fat on postprandial substrate oxidation and on carbohydrate and fat balances. *Journal of Clinical Investigation*, 76, 1019–1024.

Lissner, L., Levitsky, D. A., Strupp, B. J., Kalarf, H. J., and Roe, D. A. (1987). Dietary fat intake and the regulation of energy intake in human subjects. *American Journal of Clinical Nutrition*, 46, 886–892.

McCarty, Mark F. (1986). The unique merits of a low-fat diet for weight control. *Medical Hypotheses*, 20, 183–197.

Romieu, I., Willett, W. C., Stampfer, M. J., Golditz, G. A., Sampson, L., Rosner, B., Hennekens, C. H. and Speizer, F. E. (1988). Energy intake and other determinants of relative weight. *American Journal of Clinical Nutrition*, 47, 406–412.

Salmon, D. M. W., and Flatt, J. P. (1985). Effect of dietary fat content on the incidence of obesity among ad libitum fed mice. *International Journal of Obesity*, 9, 443–449.

Sims, E. A. H. (1986). Energy balance in human beings: The problem of plentitude. In *Vitamins and Hormones*, Vol. 43. San Diego/Orlando/New York: Academic Press.

APPENDIX B

ROUNDING OUT YOUR T-FACTOR FITNESS PROGRAMME

Cardiovascular fitness is only part of the fitness picture. A total physical activity programme also includes flexibility, and muscular strength and endurance.

First, let's talk about flexibility.

Stretching loosens you up before a walk or a jog, and cools you down after vigorous exercise. A good stretching routine works the most important areas of the body for active people: calves, hamstrings (the muscles at the rear of your legs), stomach and lower back. The T-Flex Routine will also address the areas where most of us hold a lot of our tension: the upper shoulders and neck, and again, the lower back.

Remember to stretch comfortably; don't push yourself to the point of pain. In time, with practice, your flexibility will increase naturally.

T-FLEX ROUTINE

This entire series of stretches takes only minutes to perform. Add to it some hatha-yoga postures if you wish for even greater flexibility, health and relaxation.

T-FLEX FOR THE NECK AND SHOULDERS

These first four movements are best performed while standing in the shower with hot water pouring down on your neck.

1. *Shoulder lift.* With head straight and neck relaxed, slowly lift your shoulders toward your ears. When shoulders are as high as

they can comfortably go, roll them back, pushing your shoulder blades gently together. Hold for about 10 seconds, then reverse your movements, rolling your shoulders forward to the starting position, then lowering them. Repeat.

2. *Neck roll.* From the same starting position as above, slowly let your neck roll forward and your head drop down, trying to touch your chin to your chest without straining. Hold for several seconds, then roll your head up until you're looking at the ceiling. Hold for several seconds, then return to starting position. Repeat.

3. *Head roll.* From starting position, facing forward, let your head slowly drop sideways to the left. Try to touch your left ear to your left shoulder; you can lift your left shoulder slightly to give yourself an added stretch. Don't strain. Return to starting position and repeat on the other side.

4. *Neck twist.* Facing forward, turn your head slowly to the left as if to look over your shoulder. Hold for several seconds. Return to starting position, then look to your right. Repeat.

T-FLEX FLOOR ROUTINE

1. *Sitting stretch.* Sit on the floor with your legs crossed. Bend forward from the hips, keeping your back relaxed but straight. Reach forward as far as you can to touch the floor with your hands. Stretch your shoulder joints as well as your hips. Hold for 10 to 20 seconds, then relax.

2. *Sitting toe-touch.* This one is good for the hip joints, calves and hamstrings. While still sitting, straighten your legs out in front of you. Bend forward from the hips, aim your toes back towards your head, and reach for your toes. Many people can only reach to their ankles or calves when they first do this exercise. If this is true of you, don't force yourself to go beyond the point of comfort. Hold the stretch for 10 to 20 seconds.

3. *Resting twist.* This will increase your lower back flexibility and relieve stiffness. Lie flat on the floor, arms straight out to the sides, legs together. Bend your right knee and place your right foot under your left knee. Keep your shoulders flat to the floor and rotate your lower body to the left, from the hips. Try to touch the inside of your right knee to the floor on your left side. Turn your head to the right and look out over your extended right arm. You can gently push your right knee toward the floor with your left hand, but don't force the stretch. Hold about 10 seconds. Do the other side (left foot under right knee, etc.).

4. *Back stretch.* This also helps relieve tension in the lower back. Lie flat on the floor, legs together. Bend your right leg and bring your right knee to your chest. Hold the knee with both hands and

press it gently toward your chest. Hold for 10 seconds, then reverse legs. Your head and shoulders can come up off the floor if you like, or you can use a pillow under your head for this and the next three exercises.

5. *Back curl.* Another excellent lower back exercise. Still lying on the floor, bring both knees to your chest, gently pressing them closer with your hands. Hold for about 10 to 20 seconds. Then go straight on to the next exercise.

6. *Ceiling stretch.* From the position you are already in from exercise 5, continue holding your right knee while grasping the big toe of your left foot with your left hand. Straighten the left leg up toward the ceiling as far as you can, continuing to hold the big toe. Hold for at least 10 seconds, then do the other leg. This works the calves, hamstrings and lower back as a unit. Return to the back curl position.

7. *Bicycle and flutter kicks.* From the back curl position, place your hands palms-down under your buttocks. With your knees about halfway to your chest, do a bicycling motion for 10 seconds (or 10 rotations). Then lower your legs straight out in front of you to within 6 inches of the floor and do flutter kicks for 10 seconds (or 10 repetitions). Repeat the bicycle motion, alternating with the flutter kicks, until you feel some strain in your stomach area. This exercise can take the place of sit-ups and is an excellent tummy toner and back exercise. *However, if you already suffer from chronic lower back pain, do not do this exercise without getting a professional's advice. Your problem may require a different stomach muscle strengthener.*

8. *Pelvic curl.* Still lying down, rest your arms flat on the floor with elbows bent and hands near your head, palms up. Bend your knees so that your feet are flat on the floor about 12 inches (30 cm) from your buttocks. Curl your pelvis so your lower back presses against the floor and your buttocks lift slightly. Hold for about 10 seconds, release, and repeat. This will relieve tension in the lower back.

9. *T-Factor 'shoulder stand'.* Simply place your legs up on a chair and relax for 30 seconds. This is good for your circulation, helps reduce swelling around the ankles, and will relieve 'drawing pains' in the legs. If you experience pain in your extremities during the night, do the T-Factor 'shoulder stand' before you go to bed. If you are already fairly flexible and don't have much weight to lose, you can do the more rigorous shoulder stand: Lie flat on the floor with your arms resting along your sides. Curl your legs up as if for the back curl, but keep rolling your torso up, placing your hands on your back to help keep your balance. Straighten your legs up toward the ceiling and hold for 30 seconds. *However, if you suffer from*

hypertension, do not do any exercise that requires you to lift your legs up over your head, as in a shoulder stand, without consulting your doctor.

T-STRENGTH ROUTINE

In recent years, strength or weight training has become more popular and equipment is more widely available than ever before in sports centres and private clubs.

Which kind is best? Well, this is almost like asking which is the best car or television set. A lot depends on personal preference. The important thing is that you should exercise each of the large muscle groups.

For women just beginning a strength-training programme with free weights, it's generally best to use 3 pound/1.4 kg weights. Beginning men can go up to 5 or 6 pounds/2.3 or 2.7 kg. After a few months, you may wish to increase the weights that you work with by 3 to 6 pounds/1.4 to 2.7 kg, but it is generally best for most people to do more repetitions with light weights than to risk injury by using heavy weights. In addition, using light weights leads to good tone, an 'alive' feeling, and nice lines without excessive bulking.

It's always a good idea to warm up with some stretching exercises before beginning any work with weights. See the previous section in this chapter on the T-Flex Routine.

T-Strength training starts by focusing on the neglected upper body, then adds a few movements for the stomach and legs. If you use free weights, such as the dumb-bells that are easy to find in a sports shop, work up to 10 repetitions with a weight you can handle. Normally a booklet will come with the weights that will show you a number of different exercises.

UPPER BODY SERIES

1. *Two for the shoulders.* Hold arms at your sides with palms facing the rear. Keeping arms straight, raise weights forward to shoulder height, move arms sideways, then return to down position, slowly and with control. Breathe normally at all times. Work up to 10 repetitions, then rest for at least one deep breath. Then, turn the weights so that your palms face your body, and raise your arms outward to the sides, up to shoulder level. Work up to 10 repetitions.

2. *Biceps curl.* Stand straight with arms at sides, palms facing forward. Curl forearms up to shoulder 10 times at a moderate pace.

3. *Triceps.* Keep elbows next to your body, bend forward at

about a 60-degree angle from the hips, and curl forearms, bringing weights up to your shoulders. Then, keeping elbows next to your body, straighten your arms out behind you. Repeat until you feel some strain and stop. This will build the muscle on the back of your arms, and help reduce the likelihood of loose skin on your upper arms if you have been losing weight.

4. *Forward, up, and out.* Standing upright, start with arms at your sides, palms facing body. Curling at the elbows, bring weights forward and up almost to the shoulders. Continuing in one uninterrupted motion, spread arms out to your sides, shoulder level, palms facing forward. Keep your arms slightly bent to avoid excessive strain. Return along the same path as you began and repeat up to 10 times.

LEG SERIES

5. *Heel lifts.* With weight at your side, go up and down slowly on your toes several times, resting about a second at the top each time.

6. *Half squats.* (If you are more than a few pounds overweight, don't use any extra weight for this exercise.) With arms at sides, feet at shoulder width, toes facing slightly out, squat down a third to a half of the way to the floor. Do not go beyond the point where your thighs are parallel to the floor, and keep your knees over your feet when squatting.

STOMACH SERIES

7. *Bent-knee sit-up.* Without weights, lie on your back with knees bent and feet close to your buttocks. Curl your head and shoulders about halfway up to your knees to begin with. (As you get stronger, try to get closer to your knees.) Roll back down. Arms can be held out in front of you to start, and then, as you get stronger, they can be folded across your chest. Ultimately, hands are held behind your head.

8. *Reverse sit-up.* Without weights, lying flat on the floor with arms at your sides, bring your heels back to your buttocks, and then lift knees to your chest, raising hips off the floor. Return to starting position and repeat several times. Breathe normally.

Finally, one of the very best strengthening exercises of all is the push-up, but it should not be undertaken until your stomach muscles are reasonably strong and until you can do a push-up resting on your knees rather than your toes. You can practice some easier versions of the push-up by pushing off against a wall until you get stronger.

As I said before, be sure to check with your doctor before beginning any new fitness programme. Then, get start-up instruction from a qualified teacher at your local club or sports centre.

215

APPENDIX C

FAT AND FIBRE COUNTER

KEEPING A DAILY FAT-GRAM RECORD

It's a good idea to record your fat-gram intake in a notebook until you are familiar with the fat contents of the foods you normally eat. After a few weeks, when you have made the required changes in your diet and committed the new knowledge to memory, recording will become unnecessary.

Simply write down the food item on the left-hand side of the page and the fat content in grams on the right. Add up each meal and stick within your fat-gram allowance:

> 20 to 40 grams per day for women
> 30 to 60 grams per day for men

You may also choose to photocopy this counter, or cut it out of the book, so that you can carry it in your pocket or bag.

Since the energy in fat is so concentrated (there is a gram or more of fat in each ¼ teaspoon of fat or oil, which equals 9 calories), accurate measurements of all items that contain fat are important.

For your additional information, this counter also lists the fibre content of various foods. However, unless you are curious, you do not need to keep a record of fibre intake. The suggested range of 20 to 40 grams of fibre per day for women and up to 50 grams for men is easily reached on the T-Factor Diet (our Quick Melt menus average about 30 grams of fibre per day). Many authorities suggest that you slowly increase fibre until you are consuming quantities that are at the high end of the suggested range.

HOW TO INTERPRET THE LISTINGS IN THE DIFFERENT CATEGORIES OF FOODS IN THIS COUNTER

The category 'combination foods' includes examples of a variety but not all, of the thousands of processed and packaged foods with different brand names. We have chosen representative items from different food manufacturers, or taken an average from several, without naming them. You should be aware that the same dish may vary greatly from one manufacturer to another. The only way to be certain of the fat content of packaged foods under different brand names is to read the nutrient labels.

Values for meat and fish, salads, soups, sandwiches and other dishes that are in reality combinations of ingredients are for typical recipes. If the values are for low-calorie recipes, the food item will be labelled 'low cal' or 'reduced cal'.

In the meat, fish, and poultry categories, values are for cooked portions, without added fat, unless otherwise specified. In some cases, where values vary according to cooking methods, the cooking method is specified. In the vegetable section 'cooked' values represent those achieved in a microwave with no added fat or by boiling or steaming in or over plain salted water.

Compared with many items with similar labels listed in this counter, T-Factor recipes contain far less fat and more fibre. Be sure to check the nutrient values given with T-Factor recipes in recording your fat intake when you use these recipes.

If an item is not listed in this counter, use the values of a similar food as an approximation.

ORGANISATION OF THIS COUNTER

The food items in the Fat and Fibre Counter are listed in the following order within the different food categories listed below.

Note

T = 1 *level* tablespoon
D = 1 *level* dessertspoon
t = 1 scant *level* teaspoon
1 cup = 8 fl oz/225 ml
½ cup = 4 fl oz/110 ml

ITEM	SERVING	FAT GRAMS*	FIBRE GRAMS*
1 Beverages			
Apple juice	6 fl oz/175 ml	0.0	0.0
Orange juice, frzn conc.	6 fl oz/175 ml	0.3	0.1
Carbonated low cal.	12 fl oz/350 ml	0.0	0.0
Carbonated with sugar	12 fl oz/350 ml	0.0	0.0
Carrot juice	8 fl oz/225 ml	0.2	nfa
Coffee, brewed or instant	6 fl oz/175 ml	0.0	0.0
Coffee, cappuccino	6 fl oz/175 ml	2.4	0.0
Coffee, français	6 fl oz/175 ml	3.4	0.0
Coffee, Viennese	6 fl oz/175 ml	2.4	0.0
Five Alive	6 fl oz/175 ml	0.1	0.0

* Fat and fibre counts vary as the manufacturers alter the composition of foods. The best and most up-to-date information is on the labels of pre-packed foods.

ITEM	SERVING	FAT GRAMS	FIBRE GRAMS
Grape juice	6 fl oz/175 ml	0.0	0.0
Lemonade, bottled	8 fl oz/225 ml	0.0	0.0
Orange drink	8 fl oz/225 ml	0.0	0.0
Pineapple juice	6 fl oz/175 ml	0.0	0.0
Soda water	12 fl oz/350 ml	0.0	0.0
Tea	8 fl oz/225 ml	0.0	0.0
Tomato juice	8 fl oz/225 ml	0.2	1.5

Alcoholic beverages

ITEM	SERVING	FAT GRAMS	FIBRE GRAMS
Beer	12 fl oz/350 ml	0.0	0.0
Egg nog	4 fl oz/110 ml	15.8	0.0
Gin/rum/vodka/ whisky	1 fl oz/25 ml	0.0	0.0
Lager	12 fl oz/350 ml	0.0	0.0
Liqueurs	1 fl oz/25 ml	0.0	0.0
Wine	1 wine-glass, 3½ fl oz/100 ml	0.0	0.0

Milk beverages

ITEM	SERVING	FAT GRAMS	FIBRE GRAMS
Buttermilk, less than 1% fat	8 fl oz/225 ml	2.2	0.0
Cocoa made with skimmed milk	8 fl oz/225 ml	2.0	0.2
Cocoa made with whole milk	8 fl oz/225 ml	9.1	0.2
Condensed whole, sweetened	4 fl oz/110 ml	14.0	0.0
Condensed skim- med, sweetened	4 fl oz/110 ml	0.3	0.0
Dried, whole	2 oz/56 g	3.6	0.0
Dried, skimmed	2 oz/56 g	0.2	0.0
Evaporated, skimmed	4 fl oz/110 ml	0.5	0.0
Evaporated, whole	4 fl oz/110 ml	10.0	0.0
Low-fat milk, 1%	8 fl oz/225 ml	2.6	0.0
Low-fat milk, 2%	8 fl oz/225 ml	4.7	0.0
Malted milk	8 fl oz/225 ml	9.9	0.1
Milk, semi- skimmed	8 fl oz/225 ml	3.5	0.0
Milk, skimmed	8 fl oz/225 ml	0.3	0.0
Milk, whole, 3.5%	8 fl oz/225 ml	8.0	0.0

ITEM	SERVING	FAT GRAMS	FIBRE GRAMS
Milkshake, choc., thick	8 fl oz/225 ml	17.0	0.8
Milkshake, van., thick	8 fl oz/225 ml	15.0	0.2
Ovaltine	8 fl oz/225 ml	8.8	0.0
Yoghurt drink (Ski Cool)	c. 7 fl oz/200 ml	0.6	nfa

2 Breads and Crispbreads

ITEM	SERVING	FAT GRAMS	FIBRE GRAMS
Breadsticks	1 piece	0.2	0.2
Breadsticks, sesame	1 piece	3.7	0.2
Bread, rich fruit w/o nuts	1 slice	3.4	1.4
Bread, nut	1 slice	7.0	0.8
Breadcrumbs, white, dry	3½ oz/100 g	1.9	3.4
Crackedwheat	1 slice	0.9	1.5
Crackedwheat, toasted	1 slice	0.8	1.5
Crackers, graham	2 squares	1.3	0.2
Crackers, graham, crumbs	½ cup	4.5	1.5
Melba toast	1 piece	0.2	0.1
Crackers, Ritz	3 crackers	2.9	0.3
Crackers, Ritz, cheese	3 crackers	2.9	0.3
Crackers, Jacobs, brown wheat	1 cracker	1.2	nfa
Crackers, Jacobs, brown wheat	3½ oz/100 g	17.6	nfa
Crispbreads, light	1 slice	0.2	0.2
Crispbreads, light	3½ oz/100 g	3.5	4.4
Crispbreads, light wholemeal, Allinsons	6 slices	0.7	2.3
Crispbreads, light wholemeal, Allinsons	3½ oz/100 g	2.8	8.8
Croissant	1 medium	12.0	0.4

ITEM	SERVING	FAT GRAMS	FIBRE GRAMS
Croutons, herb-seasoned	1 T	2.0	0.2
Crumpets, w/o butter	1 crumpet	0.5	0.6
Currant loaf	3½ oz/100 g (2 to 3 slices)	3.4	1.7
French toast, home-made	1 slice	6.7	0.3
Fruit/nut cake/ bread from mix	1 slice, 1/16 loaf	5.4	0.8
Hovis	3½ oz /100 g (about 2 slices)	2.2	4.6
Maltbread	3½ oz/100 g (about 2 slices)	3.3	nfa
Mixed grain	1 slice	0.9	1.4
Mixed grain, toasted	1 slice	0.9	1.4
Muffin, American, commercial	1 large	10.3	0.8
Oatcakes	1 oatcake	2.31	0.4
Oatcakes	3½ oz/100 g	18.5	3.5
Pitta bread	6"/15 cm pocket	1.0	1.5
Fruit	1 slice	0.7	0.9
Fruit, toasted	1 slice	0.7	0.9
Rice cakes	2	0.6	0.2
Roll, brown, crusty	3½ oz/100 g (2 to 3 rolls)	3.2	5.9
Roll, brown, soft	3½ oz/100 g (2 to 3 rolls)	6.4	5.4
Roll, white, crusty	3½ oz/100 g (2 to 3 rolls)	3.2	3.1
Roll, white, soft	3½ oz/100 g (2 to 3 rolls)	7.3	2.9
Roll, starch reduced	3½ oz/100 g	4.1	2.0
Roll, rye	1 roll	1.6	2.2
Roll, rye, dark, hard	1 roll	1.0	2.2
Roll, rye, light, hard	1 roll	1.0	2.1
Roll, sesame seed	1 roll	2.1	0.8
Roll, wheat	1 roll	1.7	0.9

ITEM	SERVING	FAT GRAMS	FIBRE GRAMS
Roll, white	2 rolls	4.0	0.6
Roll, wholewheat, home-made	1 roll	1.0	2.0
Rolls, part-baked	1 roll	2.2	0.4
Rolls, hotdog	1 roll	2.1	0.7
Rolls, white, home-made	1 roll	3.1	0.5
Rusks, Krisprolls	1 rusk	0.7	0.6
Rusks, Krisprolls	3½ oz/100 g	7.0	6.0
Rye bread	1 slice	0.9	1.5
Rye bread, toasted	1 slice	0.9	1.5
Rye bread, pumpernickle	1 slice	0.8	1.3
Rye bread, pumpernickle, toasted	1 slice	1.1	1.3
Ryvita, dark	1 slice	0.2	1.3
Sodabread	3½ oz/100 g (about 2 slices)	2.3	2.3
Stuffing, bread, from mix	4 oz/110 g	12.2	0.2
Taco/tostada shells	1 shell	2.2	0.2
Tortilla, cornmeal	1 medium	1.1	0.6
Tortilla, flour	1 large	3.8	1.3
Wheat	1 slice	1.0	0.7
Wheat, toasted	1 slice	0.9	0.7
Wheatberry	1 slice	1.1	1.4
White	1 slice	0.8	0.4
White, buttermilk	1 slice	0.8	0.4
White, home-made	1 slice	1.2	0.4
White, home-made, toasted	1 slice	1.2	0.4
White, bought	3½ oz/100 g (about 3 slices)	1.7	2.7
White, fried	3½ oz/100 g (about 2 slices)	37.2	2.2
Wholemeal, bought	3½ oz/100 g (about 3 slices)	2.7	8.5
Whole-wheat	1 slice	0.8	1.4
Whole-wheat, home-made	1 slice	1.0	1.8

ITEM	SERVING	FAT GRAMS	FIBRE GRAMS
Wholewheat, home-made, toasted	1 slice	1.0	1.8
Wholewheat, toasted	1 slice	0.8	1.8

3 Flours

ITEM	SERVING	FAT GRAMS	FIBRE GRAMS
Arrowroot	1 D	0.0	0.0
Barley four	1 D	0.1	0.1
Brown flour, 85%	3½ oz/100 g	2.0	7.5
Buckwheat flour	4 oz/110 g	1.3	6.1
Carob flour	4 oz/110 g	2.0	10.8
Cornflour	1 D	0.0	0.0
Cornmeal/ maizemeal	5½ oz/160 g	0.8	5.4
Rice flour	4 oz/110 g	0.4	0.0
Rye flour, light	3½ oz/100 g	1.5	10.4
Soya flour	3½ oz/100 g	12.0	2.2
White bread flour	3½ oz/100 g	1.2	3.0
White flour, cakemaking	3½ oz/100 g	1.2	3.4
White self-raising flour	3½ oz/100 g	1.2	3.7
Wholemeal flour, 100%	3½ oz/100 g	2.0	9.6

4 Cereals
Cold

ITEM	SERVING	FAT GRAMS	FIBRE GRAMS
All Bran	small: c. 1 oz/30 g	1.5	8.5
Alpen	small: c. 1 oz/30 g	1.5	2.5
Bran Flakes	small: c. 1 oz/30 g	1.0	4.5
Branwheat 100%	small: c. 1 oz/30 g	1.4	12.1
Cornflakes	small: c. 1 oz/30 g	0.2	0.3
Grapenuts	small: c. 1 oz/30 g	0.8	1.8
Jordans original	small: c. 1 oz/30 g	2.4	6.0
Muesli	small: c. 1 oz/30 g	1.9	1.9
Puffed Wheat	small: c. 1 oz/30 g	0.4	3.9
Rice Krispies	small: c. 1 oz/30 g	0.3	0.2
Shredded Wheat	2 biscuits	1.0	4.3
Special K	small: c. 1 oz/30 g	0.1	1.4
Sugar Puffs	small: c. 1 oz/30 g	0.2	1.5

ITEM	SERVING	FAT GRAMS	FIBRE GRAMS
Weetabix	3½ oz/100 g	2.0	12.9
Weetabix	2 biscuits	0.7	4.8
Wheat germ, toasted	3 T	3.0	4.0

Cooked

Porridge, home-made	3½ oz/100 g	0.9	0.8
Ready Brek (raw)	c. 1 oz/30 g	2.2	1.4

5 Cheese

Blue	1 oz/28 g	8.2	0.0
Brie	1 oz/28 g	7.9	0.0
Cheddar	1 oz/28 g	9.4	0.0
Cottage cheese, 1% fat (diet)	4 oz/110 g	1.0	0.0
Cottage cheese, 2% fat (ord)	4 oz/110 g	3.0	0.0
Cottage cheese with cream	4 oz/110 g	5.0	0.0
Cream cheese	1 oz/28 g (2 D)	9.9	0.0
Cream cheese, 'lite'	1 oz/28 g (2 D)	7.0	0.0
Feta	1 oz/28 g	6.0	0.0
Gouda	1 oz/28 g	7.8	0.0
Mozzarella	1 oz/28 g	6.1	0.0
Mozzarella, part skim	1 oz/28 g	4.5	0.0
Parmesan, grated	1 D	1.5	0.0
Processed	1 oz/28 g	7.0	0.0
Ricotta, low fat	4 oz/110 g	9.8	0.0
Ricotta, whole milk	4 oz/110 g	16.1	0.0
Roquefort	1 oz/28 g	8.7	0.0
Swiss	1 oz/28 g	7.8	0.0

6 Combination Foods

Beef pie	8 oz/225 g	32.9	0.9
Beef stew, tinned	8 oz/225 g	13.0	0.0
Beef stroganoff	8 oz/225 g	44.4	0.8
Beef veg stew, home-made	8 oz/225 g	10.5	1.0

ITEM	SERVING	FAT GRAMS	FIBRE GRAMS
Cauliflower cheese, home-made	7 oz/200 g	16.0	nfa
Cannelloni, meat & cheese	1 helping	29.3	0.6
Cheese pudding, home-made	7 oz/200 g	21.6	nfa
Cheese soufflé, home-made	7 oz/200 g	38.0	nfa
Chicken & rice, home-made	8 oz/225 g	14.6	0.0
Chicken à la king, home-made	8 oz/225 g	14.3	nfa
Chicken and veg stir-fry	1 cup	6.9	3.2
Chicken fricassee, home-made	7 oz/200 g	18.6	0.0
Chicken pie	8 oz/225 g	25.0	0.0
Chicken, cold, dressed	4 oz/110 g	21.0	0.3
Chow mein, chicken	8 oz/225 g	4.0	0.0
Chop suey, beef, home-made	1 cup	17.0	1.3
Chow mein, home-made	1 cup	4.0	0.7
Corned beef hash	1 cup	29.3	2.0
Curry w/o meat	1 cup	6.6	1.7
Aubergine Parmesan, fried version	1 cup	24.0	3.0
Lasagne	1 serving	19.3	1.5
Macaroni and cheese, home-made	3½ oz/100 g	9.7	0.2
Meatloaf	1 slice, 2½ oz/70 g	16.3	0.3
Pizza, w/o cheese	1 piece (150 kcal)	5.4	0.0
Pizza, cheese and tomato	3½ oz/100 g	11.5	0.9
Quiche Lorraine, home-made	3½ oz/100 g	28.1	0.0
Ratatouille	½ cup	7.4	1.5

ITEM	SERVING	FAT GRAMS	FIBRE GRAMS
Sandwich, club	1	20.8	1.2
Sandwich, corned beef on rye	1	10.8	0.2
Sandwich, cheese & jam	1	16.0	0.1
Sandwich, egg salad, white	1	12.5	0.3
Sandwich, ham & mayo, white	1	15.4	0.1
Sandwich, ham salad on white	1	16.9	0.4
Sandwich, r. beef on white	1	24.5	0.1
Sandwich, tuna salad on white	1	14.2	0.1
Sandwich, turkey & mayo, white	1	18.4	0.1
Spaghetti, meat sce	1 cup	16.7	0.7
Sweet & sour pork	12 fl oz/330 ml measure	21.7	0.5
Tuna noodle casserole	1 cup	11.8	0.0
Tuna salad w/mayo	½ cup	16.3	0.4
Welsh rarebit, home-made	3½ oz/100 g	23.6	nfa

7 Desserts, Cakes, Puddings and Biscuits

ITEM	SERVING	FAT GRAMS	FIBRE GRAMS
Apple crumble, home-made	1¾ oz/50 g	3.5	1.2
Apple pie, pastry top only	1¾ oz/50 g	3.8	1.1
Banana split	1	15.0	0.1
Bread and butter p/ing, home-made	3½ oz/100 g	7.8	0.6
Brownies, choc, plain	1 small	5.0	0.0
Brownies, choc w/nuts & icing	1 small	8.5	0.1
Cake, angel food	1/12 cake	0.2	0.1

ITEM	SERVING	FAT GRAMS	FIBRE GRAMS
Cake, banana	1/12 cake	11.0	0.0
Cake, carrot, w/o nuts	1/12 cake	11.0	0.0
Cake, chocolate	1/12 cake	11.0	0.6
Cake, lemon	1/12 cake	11.0	0.0
Cake, pineapple upside-down	1 (2½"/6 cm square)	9.2	0.2
Cake, pound	1/12 cake	9.0	0.0
Cake, sponge	1/12 cake	3.1	0.5
Cake, Victoria sponge	1/12 cake	13.2	0.5
Cheesecake	1/8 pie	28.0	0.2
Christmas pudding, home-made	3½ oz/100 g	11.6	2.0
Cream puff w/ custard	1	14.6	0.0
Cupcake, choc w/ icing	1 small	4.5	0.1
Cupcake, yellow w/icing	1 small	6.0	0.1
Custard, made w/ powder	3½ oz/100 g	4.4	0.0
Custard, egg	3½ oz/100 g	6.0	0.0
Danish pastry	1 medium	18.0	0.7
Danish pastry, fruit	1 medium	5.5	0.4
Danish pastry, plain	1 medium	8.8	0.2
Doughnut	1	14.0	nfa
Dumpling, apple	1	17.0	0.0
Eclair w/choc icing & custard filling	1	15.4	0.0
Eclair w/choc icing & cream	1	20.7	0.0
Fruitcake	1 (2"/5 cm square)	6.2	0.2
Jelly, ordinary or low-cal	4 fl oz/110 ml	0.0	0.0
Gingerbread	1 piece (2½"/6 cm square)	12.9	0.1
Granola/muesli bar	1 bar	5.0	0.2

ITEM	SERVING	FAT GRAMS	FIBRE GRAMS
Ice-cream cone (cone only)	1	0.3	0.0
Ice-cream, dairy	1 (3½ oz/100 g)	6.6	0.0
Ice-cream, non-dairy	1 (3½ oz/100 g)	8.2	0.0
Icing, choc fudge	for 1/12 cake	5.5	0.0
Jam tarts, home-made, shortcrust	3½ oz/100 g (approx. 2)	14.9	1.7
Lemon meringue pie	1¾ oz/50 g	7.3	0.3
Meringues, w/out cream		0.0	0.0
Mince pies, home-made, shortcrust	3½ oz/100 g (approx. 2)	20.7	2.9
Pastry, flaky, white	3½ oz/100 g (cooked)	40.5	2.0
Pastry, shortcrust, white	3½ oz/100 g (cooked)	33.2	2.1
Rock cakes, home-made	3½ oz/100 g (approx. 2)	5.4	1.4
Pancakes (English style)	1¾ oz/50 g (approx. 2)	8.1	0.4
Queen of puddings	3½ oz/100 g	7.9	0.3
Scones, white, home-made	1¾ oz/50 g	7.3	1.0
Sorbet	8 fl oz/225 ml	0.0	0.0
Shortbread, home-made	1 piece	4.3	0.3
Snack pie, fruit	1 pie	20.2	0.0
Snoballs	1 cake	4.8	0.0
Suet pudding, steamed	1¾ oz/50 g	9.0	0.5
Treacle tart	3½ oz/100 g (2 slices)	14.0	1.2
Trifle	1¾ oz/50 g	3.0	nfa
Yoghurt, frzn, low-fat	8 fl oz/225 ml	8.0	0.0
Yoghurt, frzn, non-fat	8 fl oz/225 ml	1.0	0.0
Custard cream	3½ oz/100 g	25.9	1.2
Digestive, plain	3½ oz/100 g	20.5	5.5

ITEM	SERVING	FAT GRAMS	FIBRE GRAMS
Digestive, chocolate	3½ oz/100 g	24.1	3.5
Ginger nuts	3½ oz/100 g	15.2	2.0
Home-made, white flour	3½ oz/100 g	22.0	1.7
Rich tea type	3½ oz/100 g	16.6	2.3
Lincoln type	3½ oz/100 g	23.4	1.7
Wafers, filled	3½ oz/100 g	29.9	1.6

8 Eggs

ITEM	SERVING	FAT GRAMS	FIBRE GRAMS
Boiled/poached	1	5.6	0.0
Fried	1 large	6.4	0.0
Omelette, plain, 3 egg	1 large	21.3	0.0
Omelette, cheese, 3 egg	1 large	40.0	0.0
Scrambled w/milk & fat	1 large	7.1	0.0
Soufflé, cheese	4 oz/110 g	18.8	0.0
White	white of 1 large	0.0	0.0
Yolk	yolk of 1 large	5.6	0.0

9 Fast Foods*

ITEM	SERVING	FAT GRAMS	FIBRE GRAMS
Cheeseburger	1	17.0	nfa
Chicken, dark meat, fried	3½ oz/100 g	21.0	0.2
Chicken, white meat, fried	3½ oz/100 g	23.0	0.1
Chips	1 portion	11.0	nfa
Chicken with chips	1 portion	35.2	0.8
Chicken nuggets	6 pieces	19.0	0.0
Coleslaw	1 portion	7.5	0.5
Onion rings	1 portion	16.0	nfa
Egg roll	1	14.8	0.1
Filet o'fish (in batter)	1	25.0	0.1

* *Note for British Edition:* These figures are given only as a general guide. Fat-gram counts will vary considerably according to the franchise outlet.

229

ITEM	SERVING	FAT GRAMS	FIBRE GRAMS
Fish (in batter) and chips	7 oz/200 g of each	40.0	nfa
Hamburger	1	9.8	0.3
Big Mac (US)	1	33.0	0.6
Hamburger, whopper with cheese	1	45–60.0	nfa
Quarter-pounder	1	21.7	0.7
Quarter-pounder w/cheese	1	30.7	0.8

10 Fats and Oils

ITEM	SERVING	FAT GRAMS	FIBRE GRAMS
Beef, separable fat	1 oz/28 g	23.3	0.0
Beef suet, raw	1 D	12.8	0.0
Butter	1 scant t	4.1	0.0
Butter	1 D	13.9	0.0
Butter	3½ oz/100 g	82.0	0.0
Chicken fat, raw	1 D	12.8	0.0
Clover spread	3½ oz/100 g	75.0	nfa
Delight low fat spread	3½ oz/100 g	39.6	nfa
Duck fat, raw	1 D	12.8	0.0
Golden Churn	3½ oz/100 g	70.0	nfa
Krona	3½ oz/100 g	70.0	nfa
Margarine	1 scant t	4.0	0.0
Margarine, reduced calorie	1 scant t	2.0	0.0
Mayonnaise	1 D	11.0	0.0
Mayonnaise, reduced calorie	1 D	5.0	0.0
Pork fat (lard)	1 D	12.8	0.0
Pork, backfat, raw	1 oz/28 g	25.4	0.0
Pork, separable fat, ckd	1 oz/28 g	23.4	0.0
Pork, separable fat, raw	1 oz/28 g	20.5	0.0
Salt pork, fried	1 oz/28 g	19.6	0.0
Salt pork, raw	1 oz/28 g	23.8	0.0
Shape, low-fat	3½ oz/100 g	39.0	nfa
Slimmer's Gold, low-fat	3½ oz/100 g	39.0	nfa

ITEM	SERVING	FAT GRAMS	FIBRE GRAMS
Turkey fat	1 D	12.8	0.0
Vegetable shortening	1 D	12.0	0.0
Willow spread	3½ oz/100 g	78.0	nfa

Vegetable Oils

ITEM	SERVING	FAT GRAMS	FIBRE GRAMS
Almond	1 D	13.6	0.0
Coconut	1 D	13.6	0.0
Corn	1 D	13.6	0.0
Groundnut	1 D	13.5	0.0
Olive	1 D	13.5	0.0
Palm	1 D	13.6	0.0
Palm kernel	1 D	13.6	0.0
Sesame seed	1 D	13.6	0.0
Soybean	1 D	13.6	0.0
Sunflower	1 D	13.6	0.0
Wheatgerm oil	1 D	13.6	0.0

11   Fish

ITEM	SERVING	FAT GRAMS	FIBRE GRAMS
Anchovy, tinned	3 fillets	1.2	0.0
Bass, saltwater	3½ oz/100 g	1.2	0.0
Bass, grilled w/ butter	3½ oz/100 g	12.8	0.0
Bluefish, baked or grilled w/o fat	3½ oz/100 g	6.5	0.0
Carp	3½ oz/100 g	4.2	0.0
Catfish	3½ oz/100 g	3.1	0.0
Caviare, sturgeon, granular	1 t	1.5	0.0
Caviare, sturgeon, pressed	1 t	1.7	0.0
Clams, tinned solids & liquid	4 fl oz/110 ml	0.7	0.0
Clams, tinned solids only	4 fl oz/110 ml	2.5	0.0
Clams, hard meat only	5 large	0.9	0.0
Clams, liquid only	4 fl oz/110 ml	0.1	0.0
Cockles, boiled	3½ oz/100 g	0.3	0.0
Cod, dried, salted	3½ oz/100 g	0.7	0.0
Cod, raw	3½ oz/100 g	0.3	0.0

ITEM	SERVING	FAT GRAMS	FIBRE GRAMS
Cod, fried in batter	3½ oz/100 g	10.3	0.4
Cod, baked	3½ oz/100 g	1.2	0.4
Cod, fresh, boiled	3½ oz/100 g	5.2	nfa
Crab, devilled	3½ oz/100 g	9.9	0.0
Crayfish, freshwater	3½ oz/100 g	0.5	0.0
Eel, raw	3½ oz/100 g	11.3	0.0
Eel, smoked	3½ oz/100 g	13.9	0.0
Fillets, batter dipped, frzn	2 pieces, approx. 8 oz/225 g	31.0	0.0
Fillets, light & crispy, frzn	2 pieces, approx. 8 oz/225 g	23.0	0.0
Fish cakes, fried	3½ oz/100 g	10.5	0.0
Fish fingers, fried	3½ oz/100 g	12.7	0.0
Fish pie, home-made	3½ oz/100 g	5.7	0.0
Flatfish, plaice, steamed	3½ oz/100 g	1.9	nfa
Flounder/sole/ dab/ grouper, raw	3½ oz/100 g	0.5	0.0
Haddock, grilled w/fat	3½ oz/100 g	6.6	0.0
Haddock, fried	3½ oz/100 g	6.4	0.0
Haddock, smoked	3½ oz/100 g	0.9	nfa
Haddock, raw	3½ oz/100 g	0.1	0.0
Halibut	3½ oz/100 g	1.2	0.0
Halibut, grilled w/fat	1 serving	8.8	0.0
Herring, grilled w/fat	1 fish, approx. 1½ oz/42 g	14.2	0.0
Herring, pickled	1 oz/28 g	6.0	0.0
Herring, raw	3½ oz/100 g	11.3	0.0
Jack mackerel	3½ oz/100 g	5.6	0.0
Kedgeree, home-made	3½ oz/100 g	7.1	nfa
Kipper, baked	3½ oz/100 g	11.4	nfa
Lobster newberg	7 oz/200 g	21.2	0.0
Lobster, cooked, plain	3½ oz/100 g	1.0	0.0
Mackerel, fried	3½ oz/100 g	11.3	nfa

ITEM	SERVING	FAT GRAMS	FIBRE GRAMS
Mackerel, raw	3½ oz/100 g	16.3	nfa
Mussels, meat only	3½ oz/100 g	2.2	0.0
Mussels, tinned	3½ oz/100 g	3.3	0.0
Octopus, raw	3½ oz/100 g	0.8	0.0
Oysters, tinned	3½ oz/100 g	2.2	0.1
Oysters, fried	3½ oz/100 g	13.9	0.0
Oysters, raw	5–8 med.	1.8	0.0
Plaice, fried in crumbs	3½ oz/100 g	13.7	nfa
Plaice, raw	3½ oz/100 g	2.2	nfa
Prawns, shelled	3½ oz/100 g	1.8	nfa
Red snapper	3½ oz/100 g	0.9	0.0
Rockfish, ovensteamed	3½ oz/100 g	2.5	0.0
Roe, cod, hard, raw	3½ oz/100 g	1.7	nfa
Roe, herring, soft, raw	3½ oz/100 g	3.0	nfa
Salmon, fresh, grilled	3½ oz/100 g	7.4	0.0
Salmon, tinned	3½ oz/100 g	12.2	0.0
Sardines in oil	8 med.	24.4	0.0
Sardines, raw	3½ oz/100 g	8.6	0.0
Scallops, frzn., fried	3½ oz/100 g	10.5	0.0
Scallops, raw	3½ oz/100 g	0.2	0.0
Scallops, steamed	3½ oz/100 g	1.4	0.0
Scampi, fried	3½ oz/100 g	17.6	nfa
Sea bass, white	3½ oz/100 g	0.5	0.0
Sea trout, grilled	3½ oz/100 g	11.4	0.0
Shrimps, fried	3½ oz/100 g	10.8	0.0
Shrimps, raw	3½ oz/100 g	0.8	0.0
Shrimps, tinned	4 oz/110 g	0.8	0.0
Skate, fried in batter	3½ oz/100 g	12.1	nfa
Smelt, tinned	4–5 med.	13.5	0.0
Sole, fillet, baked w/o fat	3½ oz/100 g	1.1	0.0
Sprats, fried	3½ oz/100 g	33.4	nfa
Squid, raw	3½ oz/100 g	0.9	0.0
Swordfish, grilled w/o fat	3½ oz/100 g	6.0	0.0

ITEM	SERVING	FAT GRAMS	FIBRE GRAMS
Swordfish, raw	3½ oz/100 g	4.0	0.0
Trout, rainbow, baked w/o fat	3½ oz/100 g	3.6	0.0
Trout, rainbow, fried	3½ oz/100 g	13.4	0.0
Tuna, albacore, raw	3½ oz/100 g	7.6	0.0
Tuna, bluefin, raw	3½ oz/100 g	4.1	0.0
tuna, tinned in brine	6½ oz/185 g	1.7	0.0
Tuna, tinned in oil	6½ oz/185 g	22.1	0.0
Tuna, tinned, white in brine	6½ oz/185 g	3.5	0.0
Tuna, tinned, white in oil	6½ oz/185 g	19.9	0.0
Whitebait, fried	3½ oz/100 g	47.5	nfa
Whiting, fried	3½ oz/100 g	10.3	nfa
Winkles, boiled	3½ oz/100 g	0.3	nfa

12 Fruits

ITEM	SERVING	FAT GRAMS	FIBRE GRAMS
Apple, peeled	2¾"/7 cm diam.	0.4	3.4
Apple, whole	2¾"/7 cm diam.	0.4	3.5
Apples, dried	½ cup	0.1	4.5
Apples, stewed, unswt.	1 cup	0.1	2.0
Apricots, dried	5–7 halves	0.3	6.0
Apricots, fresh	3 med (about 12 per pound/450 g)	0.4	1.5
Avocado	1 large (about 8 oz/225 g)	30.0	3.7
Banana	1 large (8¾"/22 cm long)	0.6	2.0
Blackberries, fresh	1 cup	0.5	7.0
Cantaloupe	½ melon, 5"/12 cm diam.	0.7	3.0
Cherries, sweet	10–12	0.7	1.5
Cranberries, fresh	8 fl oz/225 ml	0.2	4.0
Dates, whole, dried	3½ oz/100 g	0.4	8.7
Figs, dried uncooked	3½ oz/100 g	0.0	18.5

ITEM	SERVING	FAT GRAMS	FIBRE GRAMS
Figs, fresh	1 med.	0.2	1.5
Figs, stewed	3½ oz/100 g	0.1	10.0
Fruit cocktail, tinned	1 cup	0.3	5.0
Grapefruit	½ med., 3¾"/9 cm diam.	0.1	0.5
Grapes, inc skin	3½ oz/100 g	0.3	0.9
Honeydew melon, fresh	¼ small	0.3	1.0
Kiwifruit, fresh	1 med.	0.3	1.5
Kumquats, raw	1 med.	0.0	0.7
Lemon, raw	1 med.	0.2	0.2
Lime, raw	1 med.	0.1	0.3
Loganberries, raw	31 fruits	0.1	0.4
Loquats, raw	10 med.	0.2	0.5
Lychees, raw	10 med.	0.4	0.2
Mandarin oranges, tinned	3½ oz/100 g	0.1	0.5
Mangos, fresh	1 med.	0.6	4.0
Melon	3½ oz/100 g	0.4	1.0
Mixed fruit, dried	3½ oz/100 g	0.5	2.9
Nectarines, fresh	1 med.	0.6	2.3
Orange, fresh	1 med.	0.2	3.8
Pawpaws, raw	3½ oz/100 g	0.9	0.0
Papayas, fresh	1 med.	0.4	2.4
Passionfruit, purple, fresh	1 med.	0.1	0.2
Peaches, fresh	1 med.	0.1	1.3
Peaches, tinned	3½ oz/100 g	0.2	1.0
Pear, fresh	1 med.	0.7	4.5
Pears, tinned	3½ oz/100 g	0.1	5.5
Persimmons, fresh	1 med.	0.1	2.5
Pineapple, fresh	1 cup pieces	0.7	3.2
Pineapple, tinned	1 cup pieces	0.2	2.1
Plum, fresh	1 med/large	0.6	2.5
Plums, tinned	½ cup	0.1	3.5
Pomegranate, raw	1 med.	0.5	0.3
Prickly pear, raw	1 med.	0.5	1.9
Prunes, dried, uncooked	3½ oz/100 g	0.4	16.1
Prunes, stewed	3½ oz/100 g	Tr	7.7

ITEM	SERVING	FAT GRAMS	FIBRE GRAMS
Quinces, raw	1 med.	0.1	1.6
Raisins	3½ oz/100 g	Tr	6.8
Sultanas	3½ oz/100 g	0.2	7.0
Raspberries, fresh	3½ oz/100 g	0.2	7.4
Raspberries, tinned	3½ oz/100 g	0.2	5.0
Rhubarb, stewed	3½ oz/100 g	0.0	2.4
Strawberries, fresh	3½ oz/100 g	0.2	2.2
Strawberries, tinned	3½ oz/100 g	0.2	1.0
Tangerines, fresh	1 med.	0.2	0.3
Watermelon, fresh	1 cup	0.2	0.5

13 Meats and Poultry

ITEM	SERVING	FAT GRAMS	FIBRE GRAMS
Beef, 7.5–12.4% fat, cooked	3½ oz/100 g	9.4	0.0
Beef, 12.5–17.4%, fat, cooked	3½ oz/100 g	15.2	0.0
Beef, 17.5–22.4% fat, cooked	3½ oz/100 g	19.6	0.0
Beef, 22.5–27.4% fat, cooked	3½ oz/100 g	26.5	0.0
Beef, 27.5–32% fat, cooked	3½ oz/100 g	30.0	0.0
Beef, brisket, lean & marb.	3½ oz/100 g	30.0	0.0
Beef, stewing steak	4 oz/110 g	40.7	0.0
Beef, mince	3½ oz/100 g	23.9	0.0
Beef, corned, med. fat.	3½ oz/100 g	30.4	0.0
Beef, cubed steak	3½ oz/100 g	15.4	0.0
Beef, fillet steak, grilled	3½ oz/100 g	9.4	0.0
Beef, flank steak, fat trimmed	3½ oz/100 g	9.4	0.0
Beef, hamburger, extra lean	3 oz/80 g patty, cooked	13.9	0.0
Beef, hamburger, lean	3 oz/80 g patty, cooked	15.7	0.0
Beef, hamburger, regular	3 oz/80 g patty, cooked	17.6	0.0

ITEM	SERVING	FAT GRAMS	FIBRE GRAMS
Beef, leg (topside), lean	3½ oz/100 g	9.4	0.0
Beef, meatballs	1 oz/28 g	5.5	0.0
Beef, meatloaf	3½ oz/100 g	15.6	0.0
Beef, meatloaf, home-made	3½ oz/100 g	12.6	0.1
Beef, neck, lean, pot-roasted	3½ oz/100 g	16.9	0.0
Beef, sirloin, steak, lean	3½ oz/100 g	9.4	0.0
Beef, rib roast	3½ oz/100 g	30.0	0.0
Beef, rib roast, lean	3½ oz/100 g	15.2	0.0
Beef, topside	3½ oz/100 g	15.2	0.0
Beef, sirloin, lean, roast	3½ oz/100 g	9.4	0.0
Beef, T-bone, lean	3½ oz/100 g	10.3	0.0
Brains, all kinds, raw	3 oz/80 g	7.3	0.0
Frog legs, cooked w/o fat	4 large, 4 oz/110 g	0.3	0.0
Heart, beef, lean, braised	3½ oz/100 g	5.7	0.0
Heart, pig's, braised	3½ oz/100 g	6.9	0.0
Heart, lamb, braised	3½ oz/100 g	14.4	0.0
Kidney, beef, braised	3½ oz/100 g	12.0	0.0
Kidney, pig's, raw	3½ oz/100 g	3.6	0.0
Lamb, chop, lean only	1 chop, approx. 2 oz/56 g cooked	8.9	0.0
Lamb, chop	3½ oz/100 g	27.0	0.0
Lamb, leg, roasted	3½ oz/100 g	14.5	0.0
Lamb, loin chop, grilled	1 chop, approx. 3½ oz/100 g	29.0	0.0
Lamb, loin chop, lean only	1 chop, approx. 2 oz/56 g	5.2	0.0
Lamb, rib chop	1 chop, approx. 2 oz/56 g	18.3	0.0
Lamb, rib chops, lean only	1 chop, approx. 2 oz/56 g	4.3	0.0

ITEM	SERVING	FAT GRAMS	FIBRE GRAMS
Liver, beef, fried	3½ oz/100 g	10.6	0.0
Liver, beef, raw	3½ oz/100 g	3.8	0.0
Liver, calf, fried	3½ oz/100 g	13.2	0.0
Liver, calf, raw	3½ oz/100 g	4.7	0.0
Liver, pig's, fried	3½ oz/100 g	11.5	0.0
Liver, pig's, raw	3½ oz/100 g	3.7	0.0
Liver, lamb, raw	3½ oz/100 g	3.9	0.0
Liver, lamb, grilled	3½ oz/100 g	12.4	0.0
Pork, bacon bits	1 D	1.0	0.0
Pork, bacon back, grilled	3½ oz/100 g	33.8	nfa
Pork, bacon, streaky, grilled	3½ oz/100 g	36.0	nfa
Pork, bacon, streaky, fried	3½ oz/100 g	44.8	nfa
Pork, shoulder blade	3½ oz/100 g	28.8	0.0
Pork, shoulder blade, lean only	1 slice	9.2	0.0
Pork, whole shoulder	3½ oz/100 g	28.0	0.0
Pork, shoulder lean only	3½ oz/100 g	11.2	0.0
Pork, ham shoulder	3½ oz/100 g	28.0	0.0
Pork, ham shoulder, lean only	1 slice, 1 oz/28 g	6.5	0.0
Pork, ham shank	2 slices, 2 oz/56 g	10.9	0.0
Pork, ham shank, lean only	2 slices, 2 oz/56 g	2.7	0.0
Pork, leg, lean only	1 slice, 1 oz/28 g	4.7	0.0
Pork, gammon ham	3½ oz/100 g	11.0	0.0
Pork, gammon ham, lean only	3 oz/80 g	8.5	0.0
Pork, hamloaf, glazed	3½ oz/100 g	14.7	0.0
Pork, loin chop, grilled	3½ oz/100 g	24.2	nfa
Pork, loin chop, lean only	1 chop, approx. 2 oz/56 g cooked	7.7	0.0

ITEM	SERVING	FAT GRAMS	FIBRE GRAMS
Pork, hand	2 slices, 2 oz/56 g	14.3	0.0
Pork, hand, lean only	2 slices	2.7	0.0
Pork, pig's feet, pickled	1 oz/28 g	4.1	0.0
Pork, sausage patties	2 patties	25.9	0.0
Pork, shoulder	2 slices	36.8	0.0
Pork, shoulder, lean only	2 slices, 2 oz/56 g	5.1	0.0
Pork, sirloin, lean, roasted	3 slices, 3 oz/80 g	11.1	0.0
Pork, sirloin, roasted	3 slices, 3 oz/80 g	21.9	0.0
Pork, spare ribs, roasted	3½ oz/100 g	30.1	0.0
Pork tenderloin, lean, roast	3½ oz/100 g	12.1	0.0
Rabbit, baked	3½ oz/100 g	5.0	0.0
Tongue, beef, etc., pickled	1 oz/28 g	5.7	0.0
Tongue, beef, etc, potted	1 oz/28 g	6.4	0.0
Tongue, beef, med.-fat braised	3½ oz/100 g	16.7	0.0
Tongue, beef, smoked	3½ oz/100 g	28.8	0.0
Tongue, sheep, braised	3½ oz/100 g	25.3	0.0
Veal, shoulder blade	3½ oz/100 g	16.6	0.0
Veal, shoulder blade, lean only	3½ oz/100 g	8.4	0.0
Veal, breast stewing meat, raw	3½ oz/100 g	25.2	0.0
Veal, breast stewed w/gravy	3½ oz/100 g	18.6	0.0
Veal, cutlet, breaded	3½ oz/100 g	15.0	
Veal, cutlet, round, lean	1 cutlet	12.9	0.0

ITEM	SERVING	FAT GRAMS	FIBRE GRAMS
Veal, flank, med. fat	3½ oz/100 g	32.3	0.0
Veal, foreshank, med. fat	3½ oz/100 g	10.4	0.0
Veal, loin chop with fat	1 chop	43.8	0.0
Veal, loin chop, lean only	1 chop, approx. 2 oz/56 g cooked	4.8	0.0
Veal, loin, med. fat	3½ oz/100 g	13.4	0.0
Veal, rib chop	1 chop	18.4	0.0
Veal, rib chop, lean only	1 chop, approx. 2 oz/56 g cooked	4.6	0.0
Veal, leg lean, roasted	2 slices, approx. 2 oz/56 g	6.1	0.0
Veal, rump, roasted	2 slices	4.8	0.0
Veal, sirloin steak	½ steak	17.4	0.0
Veal, sirloin steak, lean	½ steak, 3½ oz/100 g	8.1	0.0
Veal, sirloin, lean, roasted	3½ oz/100 g	5.9	0.0
Venison, roasted	3½ oz/100 g	2.2	0.0
Whale meat, raw	3½ oz/100 g	7.5	0.0

Poultry

ITEM	SERVING	FAT GRAMS	FIBRE GRAMS
Chicken, breast w/skin, roasted	½ breast	7.6	0.0
Chicken, breast, w/o skin, roasted	½ breast	3.1	0.0
Chicken, breast, w/skin, fried	½ breast	8.7	0.0
Chicken, breast, w/o skin, fried	½ breast	4.1	0.0
Chicken, gizzard, simmered	3½ oz/100 g	3.7	0.0
Chicken, heart, simmered	3½ oz/100 g	7.9	0.0
Chicken, leg, w/o skin, roasted	1 leg	2.5	0.0
Chicken, leg, w/skin, fried	1 leg	6.7	0.0

ITEM	SERVING	FAT GRAMS	FIBRE GRAMS
Chicken, leg, w/skin, roasted	1 leg	5.8	0.0
Chicken, liver, simmered	3½ oz/100 g	5.5	0.0
Chicken, thigh, w/o skin, roasted	1 thigh	5.7	0.0
Chicken, thigh, w/skin, fried	1 thigh	9.3	0.0
Chicken, thigh, w/skin, roasted	1 thigh	9.6	0.0
Chicken, wing, w/skin, fried	1 wing	7.1	0.0
Chicken, wing, w/skin, roasted	1 wing	6.6	0.0
Duck, w/o skin, roasted	3½ oz/100 g	11.2	0.0
Duck, w/skin, roasted	3½ oz/100 g	28.4	0.0
Pheasant, w/o skin, raw	3½ oz/100 g	3.6	0.0
Quail, w/o skin, raw	3½ oz/100 g	4.5	0.0
Turkey, breast, barbecued	3½ oz/100 g	5.0	0.0
Turkey, breast, smoked	3½ oz/100 g	4.0	0.0
Turkey mince	3½ oz/100 g	14.0	0.0
Turkey, patties	1 patty, 4 oz/110 g cooked	16.9	0.0
Turkey, w/o skin, roasted	3½ oz/100 g	5.0	0.0
Turkey, w/skin, roasted	3½ oz/100 g	9.7	0.0

Processed Meats

ITEM	SERVING	FAT GRAMS	FIBRE GRAMS
Black pudding, fried	1 oz/28 g	6.1	nfa
Chicken roll	1 oz/28 g	1.3	0.0
Corned beef, jellied	1 oz/28 g	2.9	0.0
Ham, chopped	1 oz/28 g	4.3	0.0

ITEM	SERVING	FAT GRAMS	FIBRE GRAMS
Ham and pork, chopped	1 oz/28 g	6.6	nfa
Hot dog, beef	1	13.2	0.0
Knockwurst/ knackwurst	1 link	18.9	0.0
Liver pâté, goose	1 oz/28 g	12.4	0.0
Liver sausage	1 oz/28 g	7.5	
Meat paste	1 oz/28 g	3.1	nfa
Pepperoni	1 oz/28 g	13.0	0.0
Salami, ckd	1 oz/28 g	10.0	0.0
Salami, dry/hard	1 oz/28 g	10.0	0.0
Sausage, Italian	1 link	17.2	0.0
Sausage, smoked	1 link	20.0	0.0
Sausage, Vienna	1 sausage	4.0	0.0
Sausages, beef, grilled	1 oz/28 g	4.8	nfa
Sausages, pork, grilled	1 oz/28 g	6.9	nfa
Spam	1 oz/28 g	7.4	nfa
Tongue, tinned	1 oz/28 g	4.6	nfa
Turkey	1 oz/28 g	4.5	0.0
Turkey breast	1 oz/28 g	1.3	0.0
Turkey ham	1 oz/28 g	1.5	0.0
Turkey roll	1 oz/28 g	1.3	0.0

Meat Products and Dishes

ITEM	SERVING	FAT GRAMS	FIBRE GRAMS
Cornish pastie	3½ oz/100 g	20.4	nfa
Pork pie, individual	3½ oz/100 g	27.0	nfa
Sausage roll, flaky pastry	3½ oz/100 g	36.2	nfa
Sausage roll, shortcrust	3½ oz/100 g	31.8	nfa
Steak & kidney pie, pastry top only	3½ oz/100 g	18.3	nfa
Steak & kidney pie, individual	3½ oz/100 g	21.2	nfa
Bolognese sauce, home-made	3½ oz/100 g	10.9	nfa
Hot pot, home-made	3½ oz/100 g	4.2	nfa

ITEM	SERVING	FAT GRAMS	FIBRE GRAMS
Irish stew, home-made	3½ oz/100 g	7.3	nfa
Moussaka, home-made	3½ oz/100 g	13.4	nfa
Shepherd's pie, home-made	3½ oz/100 g	6.1	nfa

14 Pasta and Rice

ITEM	SERVING	FAT GRAMS	FIBRE GRAMS
Macaroni, cooked	1 cup	0.8	1.1
Noodles, chow mein	½ cup	8.0	nfa
Noodles, egg	1 cup	2.5	1.4
Noodles, manicotti	1 cup	0.4	0.7
Noodles, rice	1 cup	0.6	1.5
Spaghetti w/tom. cheese sauce	1 cup	4.0	0.6
Spaghetti, plain	1 cup	0.7	0.6
Spaghetti, w/tom. sauce	1 cup	2.5	0.7
rice, brown	4 oz/110 g	0.6	1.8
rice, fried	4 oz/110 g	7.2	1.0
rice, long grain & wild	4 oz/110 g	2.1	1.9
rice, pilaf	4 oz/110 g	7.0	0.8
rice, white, boiled	3½ oz/100 g	0.3	0.8

15 Salad Dressings

ITEM	SERVING	FAT GRAMS	FIBRE GRAMS
Blue cheese	1 D	8.0	0.0
Caesar	1 D	7.0	0.0
French	1 D	6.4	0.1
Hellmans reduced-calorie	3½ oz/100 g	29.5	nfa
Hellmans reduced-calorie	1 T	4.4	nfa
Italian	1 D	7.1	0.0
Oil & vinegar	1 D	7.5	0.0
Salad cream, Heinz	3½ fl oz/100 ml	27.8	nfa
Salad cream, Heinz	1 D	2.9	nfa
Salad cream, Weight Watchers	3½ fl oz/100 ml	8.3	nfa

ITEM	SERVING	FAT GRAMS	FIBRE GRAMS
Salad cream, Weight Watchers	1 D	0.9	nfa
Thousand Island	1 D	5.6	0.3

16 Sauces

ITEM	SERVING	FAT GRAMS	FIBRE GRAMS
Barbecue	1 D	0.3	0.1
Ketchup, tomato	1 D	0.1	0.0
Gravy, home-made	3 T	14.0	0.0
Hollandaise	3 T	18.5	0.0
Horseradish, raw	1 D	0.0	0.2
Mayonnaise, home-made	1 D	9.9	0.0
Sour cream sauce	3 T	11.9	0.0
Soy sauce	1 D	0.0	0.0
Sweet & sour sauce	3 T	0.2	0.0
Taco sauce	2 t	0.0	0.0
Tartar sauce	1 D	7.9	0.0
Teriyaki sauce	1 D	0.0	0.0
Tabasco	1 D	0.0	0.0
White sauce, medium	2 D	4.1	0.0
White sauce, thick	2 D	5.2	0.0
White sauce, thin	2 D	2.6	0.0
Worcestershire	1 D	0.0	0.0

See also Seasonings

Sweet Sauces

ITEM	SERVING	FAT GRAMS	FIBRE GRAMS
Choc fudge topping	1 D	1.9	0.4
Choc syrup	1 D	0.2	0.1
Custard	2 D	0.8	nfa
Fruit topping	1 D	0.0	0.0
Hard sauce	1 D	2.8	0.0
White sauce, home-made	2 D	2.6	0.0

17 Seasonings, Pickles, Flavourings and Baking Aids

ITEM	SERVING	FAT GRAMS	FIBRE GRAMS
Allspice, ground	1 t	0.3	0.3
Anise seed	1 t	0.3	0.3
Basil	1 t	0.1	0.3

ITEM	SERVING	FAT GRAMS	FIBRE GRAMS
Caraway	1 t	0.3	0.3
Celery seed	1 t	0.5	0.2
Chilli powder	1 t	0.4	0.6
Cinnamon	1 t	0.1	0.6
Cloves	1 t	0.4	0.2
Cumin	1 t	0.5	0.2
Curry powder	1 t	0.3	0.3
Dill seed	1 t	0.3	0.4
Dill weed, dried	1 t	0.0	0.1
Fennel seed	1 t	0.3	0.3
Garlic powder	1 t	0.0	0.1
Ginger	1 t	0.1	0.1
Mustard powder	1 t	0.6	nfa
Nutmeg, ground	1 t	0.8	0.1
Onion powder	1 t	0.0	0.1
Oregano	1 t	0.2	0.2
Paprika	1 t	0.3	0.4
Parsley	1 t	0.1	0.1
Pepper, black	1 t	0.1	0.3
Pepper, red/ cayenne	1 t	0.3	0.5
Poppy seed	1 t	1.2	0.2
Sage	1 t	0.1	0.1
Salt	1 t	0.0	0.0
Salt substitute	1 t	0.0	0.0
Tarragon	1 t	0.1	0.1
Thyme	1 t	0.1	0.3
Bovril	1 D	Tr	nfa
Chocolate, baking	1 oz/28 g	15.0	0.7
Cocoa powder	1 oz/28 g	6.0	nfa
Marmite	1 t	Tr	nfa
Olives, black	2 large	4.0	0.3
Olives, Greek	3 med.	7.1	0.8
Olives, green	2 med.	1.6	0.2
Oxo cubes	1	Tr	nfa
Pickle relish	1 D	0.1	0.2
Pickles, bread & butter	4 slices	0.1	0.1
Pickles, dill or kosher	1 large	0.2	0.5
Pickles, sour	1 large	0.2	0.5

ITEM	SERVING	FAT GRAMS	FIBRE GRAMS
Pickles, sweet	1 large	0.4	0.5
Vinegar	1 D	0.0	0.0
Yeast	1 D	0.1	0.0

18 Snacks: Nuts and Nibbles

ITEM	SERVING	FAT GRAMS	FIBRE GRAMS
Almonds	12–15 nuts, 2 D	10.0	1.9
Almonds, roasted, salted	1 oz/28 g (approx. 3 D)	16.2	2.7
Almonds, salted	12–15 nuts, 2 D	10.0	1.9
Brazil nuts	4 med.	11.5	1.3
Cashews, roasted	6–8 nuts, 2 D	7.8	1.5
Chestnuts, fresh	3 small	7.9	1.0
Coconut, dried, shredded	1 oz/28 g (4 T)	9.2	0.6
Hazelnuts (filberts)	10–12 nuts, 2 D	10.6	1.0
Macadamia nuts, roasted	6 med., 2 D	12.3	0.9
Mixed nuts	8–12 nuts, 2 D	10.0	1.6
Peanut, butter	1 D	7.3	0.7
Peanuts, raw w/o skins	1 oz/28 g, 3 D	15.0	2.7
Peanuts, raw w/skin	1 oz/28 g, 3 D	15.0	2.9
Peanuts, roasted	1 oz/28 g, 3 D	15.0	2.7
Peanuts, roasted w/skin, salted	1 oz/28 g, 3 D	15.0	2.7
Pecans	12 halves, 2 D	9.1	1.0
Pistachios	30 nuts, 2 D	8.0	1.2
Trail mix	2 D	5.1	1.2
Walnuts, black	8–10 halves, 2 D	7.7	0.7
Walnuts	8–15 halves, 2 D	8.7	0.8
Walnuts, chopped	1 D	4.8	0.5
Pumpkin seeds	2 D	8.0	1.1
Sesame seeds	2 D	8.9	1.3
Sunflower, kernels	2 D	8.7	1.1
Cheddars	1 biscuit	1.3	nfa
Cheddars	3½ oz/100 g	34.0	nfa
Cheese nibbles	1 oz/28 g (pack)	10.0	3.1
Cheese nibbles	3½ oz/100 g	36.0	11.0
Crisps, average	1 oz/28 g (pack)	11.2	0.5

ITEM	SERVING	FAT GRAMS	FIBRE GRAMS
Crisps, His Nibs	¼ oz/7.5 g (pack)	2.3	0.8
Crisps, His Nibs	3½ oz/100 g	30.3	11.9
Jacket crisps	1 oz/28 g (pack)	9.5	3.4
Jacket crisps	3½ oz/100 g	34.0	12.2
Lower-fat crisps, KP	3½ oz/100 g	25.0	13.0
Popcorn, sugar-coated	1 cup	1.2	0.3
Popcorn, air-popped	1 cup	0.2	0.3
Popcorn, microwave	1 cup	2.0	0.3
Popcorn, micro-wave with butter	1 cup	3.5	0.3
Popcorn, popped with oil	1 cup	2.0	0.3
Pork rinds, fried	1 oz/28 g (pack)	9.3	0.2
Pretzels	1 oz/28 g (pack)	1.0	0.1
Ritz	1 biscuit	0.8	nfa
Ritz	3½ oz/100 g	23.6	nfa
Tortilla chips	1 oz/28 g (pack)	7.8	0.4
Tuc	1 biscuit	1.4	nfa
Tuc	3½ oz/100 g	28.0	nfa

19 Soups

ITEM	SERVING	FAT GRAMS	FIBRE GRAMS
Asparagus, cream of, w/milk	1 cup	8.2	0.7
Asparagus, cream of, w/water	1 cup	4.1	0.7
Beef consommé	1 cup	0.5	0.5
Tinned vegetable, w/meat	1 cup	3.0	2.0
Tinned vegetable type, w/o meat	1 cup	2.0	2.0
Chicken, cream of	1 cup	9.5	nfa
Chicken noodle	1 cup	11.2	nfa
Chicken consommé	1 cup	1.4	0.2
Consommé, w/ gelatin	1 cup	0.0	0.4

ITEM	SERVING	FAT GRAMS	FIBRE GRAMS
Lentil, home-made, w/ham	1 cup	9.2	5.5
Minestrone, chunky	1 cup	2.8	0.6
Mushroom, cream of, w/milk	1 cup	13.6	0.3
Mushroom, cream of, w/water	1 cup	9.0	0.5
Onion	1 cup	1.7	0.5
Onion, french, w/o cheese	1 cup	5.8	0.2
Oxtail	1 cup	4.2	nfa
Pea, green	1 cup	2.9	1.7
Tomato, cream of	1 cup	8.2	nfa
Tomato, rice, w/ water	1 cup	2.7	0.6
Veg, w/beef, bouillon	1 cup	1.9	0.7
Veg, chunky	1 cup	3.7	1.2
Slim-a'-Soup, Batchelors, made w/water	7 oz/200 g	1.2	nfa
Weight Watchers, Heinz			
Mediterranean tomato	10½ oz/295 g (tin)	1.2	nfa
	3½ oz/100 g	0.4	nfa
Vegetable and beef	10½ oz/295 g (tin)	0.6	nfa
	3½ oz/100 g	0.2	nfa

20 Sweeteners and Sweet Spreads

ITEM	SERVING	FAT GRAMS	FIBRE GRAMS
Candied fruit	1 oz/28 g	0.1	0.5
Fruit butter	1 D	0.2	0.2
Honey	1 D	0.0	0.0
Jam, all varieties	1 D	0.1	0.1
Jelly, all varieties	1 D	0.0	0.0
Marmalade, citrus	1 D	0.1	0.1
Molasses	1 D	0.0	0.0
Sugar, all varieties	1 D	0.0	0.0
Sugar substitutes	1 t	0.0	0.0
Syrup, all varieties	1 D	0.0	0.0

ITEM	SERVING	FAT GRAMS	FIBRE GRAMS
21 Sweets and Chocolate Bars			
Boiled	1 oz/28 g	Tr	nfa
Butterscotch	1 oz/28 g	2.0	0.0
Choc chips	3 T	12.2	1.2
Choc chips, milk	3 T	11.0	0.1
Fudge, choc	1 oz/28 g	3.4	0.1
Fudge, choc w/nuts	1 oz/28 g	4.9	0.1
Gum drops	28 pieces	0.2	0.0
Jelly beans	10 pieces	0.0	0.0
Life Savers	5 pieces	0.1	0.0
Liquorice Allsorts	1 oz/28 g	0.6	nfa
M&Ms	1.89 oz/55 g	10.0	0.0
M&Ms, peanut	1.67 oz/46 g	12.0	0.0
Marshmallow	1 large	0.0	0.0
Mints	14 pieces	0.6	0.0
Opal fruits	1 tube	3.5	nfa
Peanut brittle	1 oz/28 g	4.4	0.0
Toffees	1 oz/28 g	4.9	nfa
Bounty Bar	1 oz/28 g	7.4	nfa
Milk choc	1 oz/28 g	8.6	nfa
Plain choc	1 oz/28 g	8.2	nfa
Kit-Kat	bar	12.8	nfa
Marathon	2¼ oz/62 g (bar)	16.4	nfa
Mars bar	2½ oz/62.5 g (bar)	10.6	nfa
Milky way	c. 2 oz/52 g (bar)	4.2	nfa
Twix	1.73 oz/50 g	6.0	0.0
Yorkie	2½ oz/69 g (bar)	20.5	nfa
22 Vegetables			
Alfalfa sprouts	3½ oz/100 g	0.6	3.0
Artichoke	1 lge base & soft leaf ends	0.2	3.4
Artichoke hearts	½ cup	0.4	2.9
Asparagus, cooked	3½ oz/100 g	0.3	1.5
Aubergine, raw	3½ oz/100 g	Tr	2.5
Avocado	1 med./large	30.0	3.7
Bamboo shoots	1 cup	0.4	2.0
Beans, baked, tinned	3½ oz/100 g	0.5	7.3
Beans, broad	3½ oz/100 g	0.6	4.2
Beans, French	3½ oz/100 g	Tr	3.2

ITEM	SERVING	FAT GRAMS	FIBRE GRAMS
Beans, runner	3½ oz/100 g	0.2	2.9
Beans, white, cooked	3½ oz/100 g	0.5	7.4
Beans, mung, cooked	3½ oz/100 g	1.0	6.4
Beetroot, boiled	3½ oz/100 g	Tr	2.5
Black-eyed peas (cowpeas)	3 rounded T	0.6	2.2
Broccoli, cooked	3½ oz/100 g	Tr	4.0
Brussels sprouts, cooked	6–8 med./large	0.3	2.8
Butter beans, cooked	3½ oz/100 g	0.3	5.1
Cabbage, Chinese, raw	2 cups	0.1	3.6
Cabbage, green, cooked	3½ oz/100 g	Tr	2.5
Cabbage, red, raw	3½ oz/100 g	0.2	3.4
Carrot, raw	1 large	0.2	1.5
Carrots, cooked	3½ oz/100 g	0.2	3.0
Cauliflower, cooked	3½ oz/100 g	0.2	1.8
Cauliflower, raw	3½ oz/100 g	0.2	2.1
Celery, raw	1 stalk	0.1	0.9
Chickpeas, cooked	3½ oz/100 g	3.3	6.0
Chillies, green	3 T	0.0	0.3
Chinese-style vegetables, frzn	3½ oz/100 g	4.7	2.8
Chives, raw, chopped	1 D	0.0	0.1
Corn on the cob	4-inch/10 cm ear	0.9	4.3
tinned kernels	3½ oz/100 g	0.5	5.7
Courgettes, raw	3½ oz/100 g	Tr	1.8
Cucumber, w/o skin	½ med./large	0.1	0.2
Endive	3½ oz/100 g	Tr	2.2
Laverbread, cooked, w/oatmeal	3½ oz/100 g	3.7	3.1
Leeks, raw	3–4 med.	0.3	1.3
Lentils, cooked	3½ oz/100 g	0.5	3.7

ITEM	SERVING	FAT GRAMS	FIBRE GRAMS
Lettuce, iceberg	1 cup	0.2	0.8
Marrow, cooked	3½ oz/100 g	Tr	0.6
Mushrooms	10 small	0.1	1.0
Mushrooms, fried-sautéed	4 med.	7.4	0.7
Okra, raw	3½ oz/100 g	0.2	3.2
Onions, fried	1¾ oz/50 g	16.6	2.2
Onions, raw	3½ oz/100 g	0.1	1.3
Parsley	1 D	0.0	0.0
Parsnips, cooked	3½ oz/100 g	0.2	2.5
Peas, green	3½ oz/100 g	0.4	5.2
Pepper, sweet	1 large	0.2	1.5
Pimentos	3 med.	0.5	0.6
Potato	1 med., baked w/skin	0.1	3.8
Potato, boiled, w/o skin	3½ oz/100 g	0.1	1.0
Potato, fried (chips)	10 pieces	7.6	1.4
Potato, mashed, instant	3½ oz/100 g	0.2	3.6
Potato, mashed w/milk & margarine	3 rounded T	4.3	1.4
Potato, scalloped	3 rounded T	4.8	1.4
Potato, scalloped, w/cheese	3 rounded T	9.7	1.4
Pumpkin, raw	3½ oz/100 g	Tr	0.5
Radishes, raw	3½ oz/100 g	Tr	1.0
Spring onions	5 med./large	0.2	3.6
Soybeans	3 rounded T	0.4	1.8
Spinach, cooked	3½ oz/100 g	0.5	6.3
Sweet potato	1 medium	0.3	7.3
Sweet potato, candied	3 rounded T	4.3	4.5
Tofu (soybean curd)	4 oz/110 g	4.8	0.3
Tomato	1 med./large	0.2	1.4
Tomato paste	3 rounded T	1.2	4.0
Tomato, stewed/tinned	3½ oz/100 g	0.1	1.2
Turnips, cooked	3½ oz/100 g	0.3	2.2

ITEM	SERVING	FAT GRAMS	FIBRE GRAMS
Water chestnuts	16 med.	0.2	1.8
Watercress	10 sprigs	0.0	0.1
Yam, raw	3½ oz/100 g	0.2	4.1

23 Yoghurts and Creams

ITEM	SERVING	FAT GRAMS	FIBRE GRAMS
Fruit-flavoured, Ski	3½ oz/100 g/100 ml	0.8	nfa
Fruit-flavoured, low-fat	3½ oz/100 g/100 ml	1.1	nfa
Shape, very low-fat	3½ oz/100 g/100 ml	0.1	nfa
Thick and creamy, Ski	3½ oz/100 g/100 ml	2.8	nfa
Fromage frais	3½ oz/100 g	7.9	nfa
Fromage frais, skimmed	3½ oz/100 g	0.4	nfa
Cornish cream	3½ oz/100 g	60.5	nfa
Double cream	3½ fl oz/100 ml	47.0	nfa
Double cream	1 D	4.8	nfa
Fresh 'n' Creamy	3½ fl oz/100 ml	6.0	nfa
Single cream	3½ fl oz/100 ml	18.0	nfa
Single cream	1 D	2.1	nfa
Sour cream	3½ fl oz/100 ml	18.0	nfa
Sour cream	1 D	2.1	nfa
Whipping cream	3½ fl oz/100 ml	38.0	nfa
Whipping cream/ unwhipped	1 D	3.5	nfa

INDEX

References to recipes are printed in **bold** type

THE ROTATION DIET
BY MARTIN KATAHN

It's simple, it's safe, it's fast and it's effects are lasting.

The famous Rotation Diet is designed to increase your body's metabolism so you can eat normally and lose weight permanently. Based on ten years of research and clinical experience at the Vanderbilt University Weight Management Program, directed by the author, this is a proven, easy-to-use, no-fail diet plan.

* Complete 21-day Rotation Diet plan menus for both men and women.
* Safeguards against binges, purging, and loss of motivation.
* Insurance against boredom and cheating.
* More than 100 recipes for balanced healthy meals.
* A guide to food shopping and preparation, snacks, beverages, and eating out.
* A list of low-fat, low-sugar foods you can eat to your heart's content.
* A special one-day water-loss diet to correct water retention.
* A four-step maintenance plan to ensure long-term success.

0 553 17353 7

THE ROTATION DIET COOKBOOK
BY MARTIN KATAHN

The Rotation Diet Cookbook shows you how to reduce fat, salt and calories in all your cooking but still produce delicious results.

Based on the principles of the diet that changed the shape of Britain and America.

Calories and nutritional information listed by each entry.

If weight loss is desired the recipes can easily be keyed to any stage of the Rotation Diet.

Invaluable for maintaining weight for maximum health and energy.

Main dishes, ideas for entertaining and . . . desserts!

Tips on cooking for one person, eating out, and meals to take to work.

0 553 17577 7

A SELECTED LIST OF NON-FICTION TITLES AVAILABLE FROM CORGI BOOKS

THE PRICES SHOWN BELOW WERE CORRECT AT THE TIME OF GOING TO PRESS. HOWEVER TRANSWORLD PUBLISHERS RESERVE THE RIGHT TO SHOW NEW RETAIL PRICES ON COVERS WHICH MAY DIFFER FROM THOSE PREVIOUSLY ADVERTISED IN THE TEXT OR ELSEWHERE.

☐ 28212 3	**The Oat and Wheatbran Diet**	*Diana & Thomas Jewell*	£3.50
☐ 17353 7	**The Rotation Diet**	*Martin Katahn*	£3.99
☐ 17577 7	**The Rotation Diet Cookbook**	*Martin Katahn*	£3.99
☐ 17274 3	**Recipes for Diabetics**	*Billie Little & Penny Thorup*	£3.95
☐ 17273 5	**The Herb Book**	*Ed: John Lust*	£4.95
☐ 17203 4	**The Complete Scarsdale Medical Diet**		
		Herman Tarnower & Samm Sinclair Baker	£2.99

All Corgi/Bantam Books are available at your bookshop or newsagent, or can be ordered from the following address:
Corgi/Bantam Books,
Cash Sales Department,
P.O. Box 11, Falmouth, Cornwall TR10 9EN

Please send a cheque or postal order (no currency) and allow 60p for postage and packing for the first book plus 25p for the second book and 15p for each additional book ordered up to a maximum charge of £1.90 in UK.

B.F.P.O. customers please allow 60p for the first book, 25p for the second book plus 15p per copy for the next 7 books, thereafter 9p per book.

Overseas customers, including Eire, please allow £1.25 for postage and packing for the first book, 75p for the second book, and 28p for each subsequent title ordered.

NAME (Block Letters) ....

ADDRESS ....

....